I0765984

The Hidden Dangers of Pet Vaccines

Revealing the Top Five Homeopathic Alternatives to Pet Vaccines

Dr. M. Kureshi

© **Copyright 2024 - All rights reserved.**

The content contained within this book may not be reproduced, duplicated or transmitted without direct written permission from the author or the publisher.

Under no circumstances will any blame or legal responsibility be held against the publisher, or author, for any damages, reparation, or monetary loss due to the information contained within this book, either directly or indirectly.

Legal Notice:

This book is copyright protected. It is only for personal use. You cannot amend, distribute, sell, use, quote or paraphrase any part, or the content within this book, without the consent of the author or publisher.

Disclaimer Notice:

Please note the information contained within this document is for educational and entertainment purposes only. All effort has been executed to present accurate, up to date, reliable, complete information. No warranties of any kind are declared or implied. Readers acknowledge that the author is not engaged in the rendering of legal, financial, medical or professional advice. The content within this book has been derived from various sources. Please consult a licensed professional before attempting any techniques outlined in this book.

By reading this document, the reader agrees that under no circumstances is the author responsible for any losses, direct or indirect, that are incurred as a result of the use of the information contained within this document, including, but not limited to, errors, omissions, or inaccuracies.

Table of Contents

Introduction

Pets are humanizing. They remind us we have an obligation and responsibility to preserve and nurture and care for all life. –
James Cromwell

The trust and unconditional love that a pet shows us make our lives wholesome in a unique way. But that trust and love is a two-way street. They give us absolute loyalty and acceptance, and as responsible pet owners, we must ensure the health and well-being of our furry companions.

Health and well-being involve providing proper diet and healthcare, preventing accidents, as well as protecting them against sickness and disease. Pet vaccinations have long been regarded as an important element in safeguarding against potentially fatal diseases and promoting a happy and peaceful living together for pets and their human friends. However, as new scientific breakthroughs occur in pet healthcare, dissenting voices emerge, challenging the conventional wisdom surrounding vaccinations.

This book is an attempt to explore alternative perspectives, delving into the controversial narrative of those who question the efficacy and safety of pet vaccines. In this brief introduction, we will discuss the history of pet vaccination and how the scenario has evolved in the present day. This will be followed by a brief description of why pet vaccines are advised, what benefits they offer, how frequently the vaccination has to be given, and the kind of pets who can receive the vaccination. Finally, we will briefly touch upon some of the harmful effects of these vaccinations, which have prompted pet owners to look for alternate ways to protect their pets against diseases, such as homeopathy. Let's begin!

Talking about pet vaccinations is a big debate in veterinary medicine right now. This is due to the dichotomy of the situation as we want to keep our furry friends safe from dangerous diseases, but there's also worry about giving them too many vaccines repeatedly in the shape of compound vaccines and their boosters.

Pets are often recommended to get annual vaccinations even though there's a growing body of science that yearly vaccinations aren't necessary for pets that are already vaccinated. Yet, many vets are hesitant to change how they do things. This might be because they don't often learn about practical clinical immunology and might not fully understand how vaccine immunity works (Becker, 2011).

From the evolving evidence we now have, we shouldn't have a one-size-fits-all approach to vaccinations anymore. For example, it doesn't really make sense to give the same amount of vaccine to tiny and huge dogs alike. There could be a weight difference of 50 lbs between large and small pets, so the vaccine dose should most certainly reflect this. It's likely that the dose might be too much for small dogs and cause adverse reactions. Even though we know the smallest amount needed for immunization, we still don't know the perfect amount for protecting against diseases (Becker, 2011).

Scientists are now certain the vaccine dosage should be based on the animal's weight. But even now, most state laws says that the rabies vaccine, which is the strongest one, has to be given in a full dose to pets of all sizes. This certainly has to be re-evaluated, with a weight dependent dose the way forward. More on this important topic later.

The History of Development and Use of Vaccines in Animals

The vaccination in animals started with farm animals but was later extended to pets.

In the 1700s, some farmers thought that cattle plague was a lot like smallpox. So, when they learned about a method called variolation (inoculation) in 1717, they tried to prevent cattle plague by inoculating healthy cattle with stuff from sick cattle. A booklet in 1757 recommended this, and many farmers in England followed it. But later, they realized it didn't work and actually killed a lot of cattle (McVey & Shi, 2010).

In 1774, in the Netherlands, a farmer named Geert Reinders tried a different version of the inoculation method. He saw that calves from cows that had recovered from the disease seemed resistant to getting sick. This might have been the first time they noticed the idea of maternal immunity. Reinders used this resistant period to inoculate six- to eight-week-old calves with discharge from the noses of recovered cows. He also found that it worked better if he did this inoculation two more times. This process of inoculation steered the way toward vaccination as we understand it today (McVey & Shi, 2010).

Foot and mouth disease (FMD) vaccines were some of the first vaccines made, starting in the late 1800s. Because of the work of researchers like Vallée (French), Waldmann (German), Frenkel (Dutch), and Capstick (British), FMD vaccines started being made on a large scale around 1950. This allowed millions of animals in Europe and other places to get vaccinated (McVey & Shi, 2010).

When it comes to pets, using vaccines has gone from being an experiment to a normal thing to do. The first vaccine for dogs was the rabies vaccine, which they tried out on dogs before testing it on humans in 1885. But it wasn't until the 1920s that rabies vaccines, which are now required by law in many places, became available to protect dogs from the disease (Becker, 2011).

In 1923, they introduced a combo vaccine, now known as the distemper vaccine, to prevent common diseases in dogs like distemper, parvovirus, and hepatitis. In the mid-1950s, vets were commonly using rabies vaccines made from brain tissue in dogs. Back then, the main biological products they used were rabies vaccines, a "viabilized" mix of canine distemper/hepatitis virus vaccine, and antisera, along with vaccines and antisera for hog cholera and erysipelas, leptospirosis bacterins, and clostridial toxoids. As time went on and the ability to develop and make vaccines got better, they started vaccinating more types of pets, including rabies for cats and vaccines for feline herpesvirus, parvovirus in cats and dogs, and feline calicivirus (Becker, 2011).

In the 1970s, there weren't many vaccines for pets. Each time a new one came out, they just added it to the same shot. There was never any testing done to see if these combo vaccines were tolerated together, and didn't have any adverse side effects.

By the 1980s, they were giving 12 or 14 different vaccines together. But an immunologist knew that wasn't a good idea. Pets getting these combo vaccines were starting to have adverse health reactions, strongly indicating that combo vaccines were harmful to pets.

In 1978, Dr. Schultz and Dr. Fred Scott came up with a plan for how often pets should get vaccinated. They said they should get shots when they're puppies or kittens, then again at one year old, and then every three years or even less after that (Becker, 2011). Their emphasis was on avoiding over vaccinating, as they suspected that was causing a host of immunological reactions.

But it took a long time for things to change. It wasn't until 1998 that the American Association of Feline Practitioners made guidelines similar to what Dr. Schultz and Dr. Scott had said 20 years earlier (Becker, 2011).

Current Status of Pet Vaccination.

When puppies and kittens are born, they get antibodies from their mothers. These antibodies protect them from many diseases for the first few months of life. They can also can stop vaccines from working properly. That's why many vets delay vaccination until the maternal antibodies have worn off.

Back in the 1970s, when extensive vaccination in pets was being introduced, vets would make a chart for litters to figure out when they could be vaccinated effectively. This chart was based on the mothers' antibody levels. By using the time it takes for half of the antibodies to go away, they could predict when the babies' immune systems would be ready for vaccines. The mother's antibodies usually wear off between about five and a half to nine weeks (Becker, 2011).

The time between when a baby animal loses its mother's antibodies and when its own immune system is strong enough is a crucial period. During this time, if the puppies or kittens catch a virus, it can potentially be dangerous. Vets figure out this time using a chart, called a nomograph, that helps them know exactly when to give the baby animal a vaccine. With this method, they can predict when the mother's antibodies won't protect the litter anymore. This way, vets can give the right vaccines at the right times and avoid giving unnecessary shots (AVMA, n.d.).

However, there are some downsides to using the nomograph. It takes a bit of time to get the results, and the mother's antibodies for different viruses wear off at different times. For example, a puppy might be protected against distemper at 8 weeks but not against parvo until 12 or 14 weeks (AVMA, n.d.).

Many pet owners today choose to work with holistic veterinarians who use single vaccines. This approach allows for a customized and ideal vaccine schedule. Single vaccines are made to protect from only one disease, as opposed to combo vaccines that are designed to protect against multiple diseases.

As cats and dogs are the most commonly kept pets and most vaccines are manufactured to prevent diseases in them, it's pertinent to view the vaccines that target those diseases.

At present, there are two main types of vaccines used for cats and dogs: **core vaccines and non-core vaccines**. Core vaccines are said to be essential for every dog and cat, while non-core vaccines are given based on the pets' lifestyle and special needs, especially if they are exposed to unusual diseases requiring extra protection.

Core vaccines for dogs include (American Animal Hospital Association [AAHA], 2022a):

- **Distemper**: A virus that attacks the nervous, respiratory, and gastrointestinal systems, especially affecting puppies.

- **Parvo**: A highly contagious virus spread through direct or indirect contact with infected feces.

- **Adenovirus**: An acute liver infection caused by canine mast adenovirus, transmitted through saliva, blood, urine, feces, and nasal discharge.

- **Rabies**: A virus causing inflammation of the brain, affecting humans and mammals, transmitted through bites from infected animals. This is the only legally required vaccine. The rest of the core vaccines can be refused by the pet owner if they choose.

Core vaccines for cats include (Dodds, 2013):

- **Panleukopenia**: A highly contagious infection affecting the nervous, immune, and gastrointestinal systems in kittens and cats.

- **Calici**: Causes oral disease and upper respiratory infections in cats.

- **Herpes**: Affecting kittens and cats, spread through direct contact with virus particles in saliva and nasal discharge.

- And **Rabies**. As for dogs, this is the only legally required vaccine. The rest of the core vaccines can be refused by the pet owner if they choose.

These diseases can be severe, with mortality rates as high as 60% to 80% in young animals. However, most vets agree that only the core vaccine, **panleukopenia**, is a must-have for indoor kitties; the rest are optional based on the cats lifestyle.

Non-core vaccines are also optional and are recommended based on certain animals' risk factors, such as their lifestyle or location. For instance, dogs living or traveling to areas with disease-carrying ticks may be advised to get vaccinated against Lyme disease. Dogs frequenting places where other dogs gather, such as boarding, daycare, and training facilities, may be recommended to receive Bordetella and canine influenza vaccine (Dodds, 2016a).

You might wonder about the benefits of vaccinating pets and why it's necessary. Vaccines are purported to activate the developing animals immune system, prompting it to create antibodies. This way, if a dog or cat encounters an infectious disease, its immune system can respond and fight it off. Traditional veterinarians emphasize that vaccinations play a crucial role in protecting pets from highly contagious or deadly diseases, enhancing their overall quality of life. Yet, holistic veterinarians take a more measured approach, preferring natural immunity and holistic health care to augment vaccines, or even replace them.

The Issue of Frequent Vaccination and Lifetime Immunity

Traditional veterinarian recommend that puppies and kittens are immunized at around three-week intervals once the maternal-derived antibodies decrease to noninterfering levels. This vaccination series is usually given every 2 weeks between the 4th and 16th weeks of life. For those with higher risks, such as certain breeds or environments, vaccinations may be administered at younger ages or more frequently. Rabies vaccination is commonly initiated at four months of age, and booster doses are often provided at one year for most vaccines. Following these immunization practices is said to ensure a strong duration of immunity, lasting at least five to seven years and even longer in some cases. General recommendations from the World Small Animal Veterinary Association suggest vaccinating every third year after the initial series, aligning with product label guidelines (Dodds, 2016a).

In the United States, the standard practice was to administer a five-way combination vaccine to puppies at 6, 8, 10, 12, 14, and 16 weeks, followed by an annual booster throughout their lives. This is now seen as excessive and possibly harmful to the young animals developing immune system.

Holistic veterinarians propose an alternate schedule, where minimal vaccinations are preferred. They prefer to let the animal's immune system mature naturally, and not overburdened with excessive vaccines, which can be counter productive and even cause harm to the animal.

Holistic veterinarians also perform vaccine antibody titers in lieu of repeated vaccinations. This is a test to measure the level of antibodies in the animal's blood before re-vaccination. If the level is already protective, the need for annual booster vaccinations can be waived.

Reasons for Pet Vaccine Hesitancy

The reason for vaccine hesitancy can be summed up in two words: **adverse reactions in pets and vaccine**

failures.

Severe side effects of vaccination include the possibility of an allergic reaction, which may occur shortly after vaccination and can affect part or all of the body, posing a life-threatening risk. Signs of such reactions include fainting or collapse, persistent vomiting or diarrhea, and difficulty breathing.

In cats, there is a serious potential reaction involving the development of a specific type of tumor at the injection site (sarcoma). These tumors may appear several months or even years after receiving a vaccine. This is known as FISS (Feline injection site sarcoma) (AVMA, n.d.).

Post-vaccination reactions can be attributed to various causes, including (AVMA, n.d.):

- Inappropriate administration of a modified-live product.

- Innate immune responses to the vaccine.

- Specific cell-mediated or humoral immune responses to vaccine components.

- The unlikely event of vaccine antigens returning to virulence, provided the vaccines are appropriately tested and licensed.

Vaccination failures may happen due to (AVMA, n.d.):

- The vaccinated patient failing to mount a sufficient immune response.

- Exposure to the infection before completing the full vaccination schedule.

- Interference from maternal antibodies.

- Mishandling or improper storage of the vaccine, including incorrect administration.

- Waning immunity, such as immunosenescence, refers to age-related deterioration of the immune system.

- Vaccine manufacturing errors, such as lack of potency due to instability, expiration, or improper storage.

The distress of witnessing your pet suffer, especially when the intention was to safeguard them, is highly upsetting. Therefore, having comprehensive information about the advantages and disadvantages of pet vaccination is crucial for making informed decisions. In the upcoming chapters of this book, you will encounter enlightening as well as disturbing details about vaccines that aim to expand your understanding and empower you to make more informed choices when it comes to your pet's health.

Chapter 1:

The Pet Vaccine Schedule

Should you consider vaccinating your pet or not? Traditional veterinarians strongly advise against completely forgoing vaccinations, as they claim unvaccinated pets face a significantly higher risk of contracting and spreading deadly diseases, with mortality rates reaching as high as 80% (Becker, 2023b). Pet owners naturally desire to ensure the happiness and well-being of their pets by safeguarding them from severe illnesses that could prove fatal. The challenge is understanding what vaccinations are truly essential and determining which ones are acceptable to skip, particularly for indoor-only pets. To navigate this, pet owners need to be well-informed about the recommended pet vaccination schedule.

This chapter discusses not only pet vaccination schedules but also sheds light on the diseases these schedules aim to protect pets from. We will explore the scientific explanations provided by veterinarians regarding the benefits of vaccinations and delve into the legal requirements associated with pet vaccinations.

It is crucial to note that animals must be in good health to receive vaccinations. Animals with a history of adverse vaccine reactions, autoimmune diseases, chronic illnesses (including organ disease, thyroid/adrenal disease, and cancer), or those taking immunosuppressant drugs should refrain from vaccination entirely.

The Scientific Rationale Vets Use to Recommend Vaccination

The endorsement of vaccinations by veterinarians is due to their purported capacity to stimulate the production of antibodies, providing crucial support to a pet's immune system in warding off potential contagious illnesses that could compromise their well-being. The process involves introducing a disease-causing organism to your dog or cat during vaccination, thereby triggering their immunity and imparting their immune system the knowledge of how to combat these diseases in the future (European Advisory Board on Cat Diseases [ABCD Europe], 2022). From a physiological perspective, scientists explain that immunity is achieved through the multiplication of specialized cells, primarily lymphocytes. These cells can either directly eliminate virus-infected cells or produce proteins that aid in the defense against the pathogens. In the case of orally administered, attenuated vaccine viruses, replication occurs in the intestinal tract, leading to the synthesis of antibodies (ABCD Europe, 2022). This preventive approach may facilitate the eradication of the virus from the local population. It's worth noting that immune lymphocytes have finite lifespans, and antibodies diminish over time (ABCD Europe, 2022).

Scientists emphasize that the purpose of vaccination extends beyond individual protection against diseases caused by bacteria and viruses; it also plays a crucial role in preventing infection and transmission within a population. Achieving vaccination coverage of around 70% or more, they say, establishes "herd immunity," serving as a safeguard against epidemics (ABCD Europe, 2022).

The main concern of pet owners is to be able to choose which vaccine to skip and which to administer. To make this decision, they need to know which diseases their pets are more likely to be exposed to, considering their lifestyle and geographical location. The vaccine schedules make a distinction between core and non-core vaccines based on the principle that some diseases can target all cats and dogs regardless of whether they are indoor-only or outdoor pets or whether they frequent boarding facilities and groomers or not. Vaccines offering protection from these diseases are put in the core category and are often recommended by traditional veterinarians.

Core Vaccines for Dogs

Several diseases, each caused by specific viruses, pose a threat to all dogs, including:

Distemper: A virus affecting the respiratory, gastrointestinal, and nervous systems of dogs.

Adenovirus: This disease targets the liver, inducing symptoms resembling hepatitis in dogs.

Parvovirus: Causing acute gastrointestinal illness, anorexia, and lethargy in infected dogs.

Rabies: A disease that attacks the nervous system, spreading through animal bites. This is legally required in almost every jurisdiction.

Additionally, your veterinarian may recommend one or more non-core vaccinations based on specific circumstances. Non-core vaccinations, is it believed, may be necessary if a particular disease is prevalent in your area or if your pet frequently travels or interacts with other dogs (Becker, 2023b).

Non-core Vaccinations for Dogs

Bordetella (kennel cough): Recommended for pets in contact with other dogs at places like boarding facilities, dog shows, dog parks, or training classes.

Lyme disease: Considered if you live in an area where Lyme disease is widespread.

Leptospirosis: Recommended if your dog spends significant time outdoors, as this disease is spread through the urine of wild animals.

Crotalus atrox: This vaccine reduces the risk of death if your dog is bitten by certain types of rattlesnakes found in California.

Influenza: Reduces the severity of canine flu symptoms if your dog contracts the illness (Becker, 2023b).

Core Vaccines for Cats

- **Panleukopenia**: A highly contagious infection affecting the nervous, immune, and gastrointestinal systems in kittens and cats.

- **Calici**: Causes oral disease and upper respiratory infections in cats.

- **Herpes**: Affecting kittens and cats, spread through direct contact with virus particles in saliva and nasal discharge.

- And **Rabies**. As for dogs, this is the only legally required vaccine.

Non-core Vaccinations for Cats

Additional non-core vaccines, which may be recommended for specific situations, include:

- **Bordetella**: While not universally needed, the bordetella (kennel cough) vaccine becomes prudent if you have multiple cats or if your feline companion occasionally stays in a boarding facility.

- **Chlamydia**: This vaccine, addressing conjunctivitis (pink eye) and upper respiratory infections, is suitable for multi-cat households and cats that frequently go outdoors. It can be administered as part of the combination vaccine or separately, depending on the circumstances (Becker, 2023b).

The Vaccine Schedule for the Most Popular Pets (Dogs, Cats)

Vaccine Schedule for Dogs

Before 2011, annual administration of core vaccines (distemper, parvo, and adenovirus) was the norm. However, updated guidelines introduced a more extended interval, allowing core vaccines to be given every three years or longer. Notably, the American Animal Hospital Association (AAHA) acknowledged that immunity persists for at least five years for distemper and parvo and at least seven years for adenovirus.

Concerning non-core vaccines, veterinarians typically discourage their use unless the risk of contracting the disease significantly outweighs the potential vaccine-associated risks (AAHA, 2022a).

The 2022 AAHA Canine Core Vaccination Recommendations are as follows:

- **Combination vaccine:** Canine distemper (CDV) + canine parvo (CPV-2) + canine adenovirus (CAV-2) + (optional) canine parainfluenza virus (CPiV)

- **Initial vaccination in puppies up to 16 weeks:** At least three doses of a combination vaccine between 6 and 16 weeks, 2-4 weeks apart.

- **Initial vaccination in dogs over 16 weeks:**

Two doses of a combination vaccine, 2-4 weeks apart.

- **Re-vaccination:** A single dose of a combination vaccine within one year following the last dose in the initial vaccination series. Subsequent boosters should be administered at intervals of three years.

As for rabies, experienced veterinarians typically recommend the first vaccine at six months, followed by legally required boosters one year later and subsequently every three years (AAHA, 2022a). Holistic veterinarians recommend a more spaced out time frame for rabies boosters, recognizing the recent scientific understanding that the antibody protection can last for 5 years or more.

Vaccination Schedule for Cats

For kittens aged 6-10 weeks, the recommended vaccination is FVRCP (feline distemper). Between 11 and 14 weeks, the vaccination schedule expands to include both FVRCP (feline distemper) and FeLV (feline leukemia). Once your cat reaches 15 weeks or older, the vaccination protocol encompasses FVRCP (feline distemper), FeLV (feline leukemia), and the rabies vaccine (AAHA, 2022a).

Moving into adulthood, cat vaccinations are administered one year after completing the kitten series. This includes a combination vaccine of FVRCP (feline distemper), FeLV for cats with potential exposure to feline leukemia (especially those unsupervised outdoors), and the rabies vaccine annually, in compliance with legal requirements (AAHA, 2022a).

It's important to note that a combination vaccine consists of feline distemper, rhinotracheitis, and calicivirus. According to the American Veterinary Medical Association and the American Association of Feline Practitioners, cats at low risk of disease exposure may not require yearly boosters for most diseases (AAHA, 2022a).

Important Considerations Before Vaccinating Pets

It is crucial to emphasize that all animals must be in good health to undergo vaccinations. If your pet is currently dealing with any health issues or has received a new diagnosis affecting their well-being, they are not eligible for the vaccination schedule, and should forego all vaccinations.

Your pet should be in overall good health. Conditions such as allergies, endocrine issues, organ dysfunction, cancer, or a history of being a cancer survivor disqualify them from receiving vaccines. Also, these points should be noted before considering vaccinating your pet.

- The vaccine targets a life-threatening disease, eliminating most non-core options immediately.

- The vaccine is considered both effective and safe, bearing in mind that not all vaccines meet these criteria, especially bacterins.

- Your pet has never experienced an adverse reaction to a vaccine. Pets with a previous vaccine reaction of any kind should not be vaccinated.

If you choose to vaccinate your pet, it is advisable to request a homeopathic vaccine detox, such as Thuja, from your integrative veterinarian. Chlorella can also aid in removing adjuvants, typically aluminum and thimerosal (mercury) (Becker, 2023c). Unfortunately, most traditional veterinarians do not offer single vaccines, so it is prudent to inspect the vaccine vial to ensure your pet is receiving only one agent at a time, known as a single use vaccine.

Interestingly, some pet owners and progressive veterinarians in countries like the Netherlands and Belgium have developed more advanced titering protocols. In these regions, many vets titrate puppies and kittens before their initial vaccines to assess the presence of maternal antibodies (Becker, 2023c). This approach allows for the precise timing of the first vaccine, followed by a titer test four weeks later to confirm adequate immunization.

The Legal Requirement to Vaccinate Pets (i.e., Rabies)

Given the lethal nature of rabies and the consequential requirement to euthanize infected pets, veterinarians strongly advise appropriately vaccinating pets with the rabies vaccine (Becker, 2018). Compliance with vaccination laws and avoiding situations where pets might encounter rabid animals are essential measures for pet protection.

Rabies, also known as acute viral encephalomyelitis, is a potentially fatal inflammatory infection affecting the brain and central nervous system. In the U.S., the primary mode of transmission to dogs and cats is through bites from infected foxes, raccoons, skunks, coyotes, or bats (Becker, 2018). As a zoonotic disease, rabies can be transmitted to humans through contact with infected animals. Once the rabies virus enters a pet's body, it multiplies in muscle cells and migrates through peripheral sensory and motor nerves to the brain and central nervous system. In dogs, symptoms typically appear three to eight weeks after exposure, while in cats, it occurs two to six weeks after exposure (Becker, 2018).

Immediate treatment is crucial for any chance of a pet's survival once symptoms manifest. If there's a suspicion of exposure, such as a fight with another animal, a bite or scratch, or contact with a potentially rabid animal, prompt veterinary attention is necessary.

The amount of rabies vaccine administered is a contentious topic among veterinarians. While many integrative vets argue against a "one size fits all" approach, stating that it poses a higher risk of rabies vaccine reactions in dogs under 40 pounds, the law mandates a uniform 1-milliliter dose for all dogs (Becker, 2018). Some states permit medical exemptions for pets who are unwell or have previously experienced adverse reactions. It is advisable to delay the first rabies vaccination until the pet reaches the maximum age permitted by law. This may be six months in some states and earlier in others. Delaying the vaccine helps prevent issues such as vaccine failure, which is more common in puppies under three months, as highlighted in a Greek study (Becker, 2018).

Experienced veterinarians often recommend administering a three-year rabies vaccine after the second rabies shot, providing protection for the remainder of your pet's life. The three-year vaccine is essentially the same as the one-year vaccine, fulfilling the legal requirements but with significantly less frequent administration (Becker, 2018). This approach reduces the number of vaccines your pet receives throughout its life, thereby minimizing the potential for adverse reactions.

Crucially, rabies vaccinations should never be combined with or given simultaneously with other vaccines. They should be administered alone, with a minimum two-week separation from all other vaccinations. A recent retrospective study highlighted that many beloved pets are subjected to over-vaccination against rabies over their lifetimes (Becker, 2018). Until city and state vaccine laws are modified to accept titers instead of vaccinations, this issue will persist as a medical concern for numerous animals.

How Long Does a Pet Vaccine Last?

Is it necessary to routinely administer parvovirus, distemper, and adenovirus vaccines?

Recent research on antibody titer testing suggests that vaccine-induced immunity against canine parvo, distemper, and adenovirus is long-lasting, particularly in senior and geriatric dogs, making these tests valuable indicators of immunity (Becker, 2011).

One study revealed that 50% of previously vaccinated elderly dogs retained protection against the three core diseases, while another concluded that vaccines provide immunity for at least five years in most dogs (Becker, 2011). **It's crucial to recognize that vaccinations do not always guarantee immunization; titer tests play a crucial role in determining if your pet is protected.** A positive titer indicates protection, but a negative result doesn't necessarily imply vulnerability. Over time, circulating antibody levels may decrease, yet the immune system retains memory to mount a response if exposed to the disease, and can produce more antibodies if needed.

Studies confirm that for distemper, parvovirus, and adenovirus, a positive titer test is a definitive indicator of protective immunity in dogs (Becker, 2011). It's important to note that these core vaccines are not legally required. While private entities like veterinary clinics or groomers may mandate them, they are not state-mandated. Many pet owners are hesitant to ask for a titer test, fearing legal consequences, but in reality, they are not breaking any laws, as there is no legal requirement to vaccinate, outside of rabies.

Legally, the only required vaccine is rabies. Unfortunately, due to mandatory rabies vaccines in most countries, **a positive rabies titer test is only legally recognized as an indication of protective immunity**

for humans, not for pets (Becker, 2011). This situation needs addressing, as laws not grounded in scientific evidence compel pet owners and veterinarians to repeatedly re-vaccinate animals already immune to rabies. These unnecessary re-vaccinations do not enhance immunity and can be harmful to some animals.

Chapter 2

The Scientific Rationale for Vaccinating Pets

In the world of responsible pet parenting, keeping them healthy involves understanding how their immune system works and how vaccinations may help. It's not just a regular visit to the vet; it's a crucial part of making sure our pets live a happy and long life. Exploring the science of pet immunology reveals interesting ways their body defends against sickness, and we'll also look into how vaccinations help in this process. Let's dive into the world of antibodies, antigens, and the ongoing science that helps protect our beloved pets from potential dangers around them.

A Simple Introduction to Pet Immunology

The study of immunology holds immense significance for veterinarians due to the longstanding impact of infectious diseases on humans, their pets, and livestock, which requires effective control measures. Immunology is a crucial field within the medical and biological sciences as it focuses on studying the immune system, which is basically the body's defense against infections. A well-functioning immune system plays an important role in safeguarding against diseases, such as autoimmunity, allergies, and cancer (Tizard & Payne, 2011).

Immunology essentially explores the science behind the body's defense mechanisms. Our surroundings are teeming with bacteria, viruses, and various potential invaders. The reason the immune system is complex is that it has to deal with many different kinds of threats (Tizard & Payne, 2011). These threats can be bacteria, viruses, and other things that could make our pets sick. To protect them effectively, the immune system has to use different ways of fighting off each type of threat. It's similar to possessing a toolkit with various tools designed for specific tasks. The immune system needs this variety to keep the pets safe from all the different things that could harm them.

The immune system can be broken down into three fundamental components: **physical barriers, innate immunity, and adaptive immunity.** These parts work together to keep us and animals safe from sickness (Tizard & Payne, 2011). Breaking it down helps us see how important the immune system is for survival. Because there are so many different things that can make pets sick in our surroundings, using just one way to protect them wouldn't work well. The immune system needs to be complex and multifaceted to defend the pets against the various threats they might encounter.

Looking at our pets and other animals we live with, like dogs, cats, livestock, and poultry, we see a lot of different species. But all these animals need a strong immune system to stay healthy. It's interesting to know that their immune systems are quite different from mice and humans. Even though most research on immunity is done with mice and humans, it doesn't always apply to our domestic animals.

Animals, just like humans, can have immune-related problems like allergies or autoimmune diseases. The immune system is a complex network in our bodies designed to protect us from diseases. It has different parts, both at a molecular and cellular level. These parts work in two ways: There are general mechanisms that are always there (innate), and specific responses that adapt to certain threats (adaptive). Studying these components is what fundamental or classical immunology is all about (Roth et al., n.d.).

The first layer of defense in our body is called innate immunity, and it's not picky—it responds in the same way to all kinds of potential threats, no matter how different they are. Innate immunity has physical barriers like our skin and saliva, as well as cells like macrophages, neutrophils, basophils, and mast cells. These components are always ready to jump into action and protect us in the first few days of an infection. Sometimes, they manage to clear the threat on their own, but in other cases, when the first defense is overwhelmed, a second layer of defense comes into play (Tizard & Payne, 2011).

The second line of defense is adaptive immunity, and it's like our body's memory system. It remembers past infections, allowing us to mount a stronger and more specific response when facing the same pathogen again. Adaptive immunity involves antibodies, which target foreign pathogens floating in our bloodstream. T cells are also part of this defense, specifically dealing with pathogens that have invaded our cells. They can either directly kill infected cells or help regulate the antibody response. (Tizard & Payne, 2011).

Understanding how a disease develops and the factors that make it harmful helps us figure out the best way to protect against it. **Often, the most effective immunity comes from recovering after having the actual disease, known as natural immunity.** Vaccination aims to mimic this natural immunity but without causing the animal to go through the illness associated with the real infection (Tizard & Payne, 2011). Science has repeatedly demonstrated that vaccine derived immunity is not as robust and protective from future exposures, as is natural immunity.

There are different types of immune responses to a pathogen (Roth et al., n.d.):

- **Humoral response**, this includes:
    - **Circulating antibodies**: These are proteins (like IgM and IgG) found in our blood.
    - **Mucosal antibody response**: Antibodies (like IgA) on mucosal surfaces such as the nose, mouth, lungs, and stomach respond to threats.

- **Cell-mediated response:**
    - ○ Involves activating different cells in the immune system, like Cytotoxic T Cells, which directly recognize and kill infected cells, and Gamma Delta T Cells, which help protect mucosal surfaces.

Knowing about how the organism causes the disease helps us identify which antigens (substances that trigger an immune response) are crucial for building a protective immune response. In simpler terms, understanding the disease's process helps us make informed decisions about what's needed for effective protection (Roth et al., n.d.).

How Vaccines Prevent Diseases and Confer Immunity According to Scientists and Vets

Let's go back to the basics of immunology to see how it connects with vaccination. In simple terms, the immune system is like our body's defense team, protecting us from harmful invaders like bacteria. These invaders have proteins and molecules called antigens, and our immune system fights back by creating antibodies.

Now, drugs can influence the immune system in different ways. One common method is *specific immunotherapy,* where a specific antigen, like in a *vaccine,* triggers a controlled immune response. This purportedly leads to effective and long-lasting immunity. Another way, called *nonspecific immunotherapy,* encourages the immune system to produce proteins that make it stronger. It can also give an overall boost to help fight off infections. In this category, we have *adjuvants added to vaccines* to make them work better. Yet, adjuvants can also cause harm, in a process known as *hyper-stimulation of the immune system.* In fact, many vaccines are made specifically reducing or eliminating adjuvants due to their troubled history of causing harm.

How Do Vaccines Actually Work?

Just like human vaccinations, pet vaccines use an agent similar to the disease-causing microorganism, known as an antigen. When this agent is injected into your pet's bloodstream, their immune system recognizes it as a threat and mounts an immune response to fight it off. This process helps your pet's immune system remember the disease, making it ready to combat it if encountered later. It usually takes about a week for your pet's body to respond to the vaccine and build immunity (AVMA, n.d.).

Scientists have created different types of vaccines for animals. In the past, vaccines were sorted based on whether they had live or dead organisms. Vaccines with dead organisms are not as good at triggering a strong immune response compared to those with live ones. To make dead organism vaccines work better, they often include extra substances called adjuvants, aiming to boost the vaccine's overall effectiveness. These killed vaccines might have the entire dead organism or just a part of it that sparks the immune response. A type 1 recombinant vaccine also falls under the category of killed vaccines.

While vaccines with live organisms are often more effective, there are challenges in making them because these live organisms can also cause disease if not modified. Attenuated vaccines are a solution—they contain altered live organisms that are less likely to cause illness. They can reproduce, prompting a strong immune response. Yet, even with these modified vaccines, there's a risk they may revert to being harmful and cause the very disease they're meant to prevent. To boost safety, type 2 recombinant vaccines, or gene-deleted vaccines, were created. They remove the specific genes that cause disease, ensuring the live organisms can generate a strong immune response but can never cause illness.

Besides vaccines, there are other ways to boost immunity against diseases. Passive immunity involves one animal producing antibodies and then passing them to another animal for immediate protection. For example, mothers naturally transfer antibodies to their offspring through the placenta and colostrum (the first milk full of essential antibodies). Antisera produced in dogs against distemper and in cats against panleukopenia also provides passive immunity. However, this type of immunity is temporary, lasting only as long as the transferred antibodies remain active, usually a few weeks.

Even after getting vaccinated, your pet may not develop immunity against the disease for which it was vaccinated. This is called vaccine failure, and it can be a result of many factor such as:

Maternal Antibodies:

When a puppy/kitten is born and feeds on its mother's milk, it gets antibodies from her. A mother passes on protection for diseases she's naturally encountered. These antibodies shield the puppy/kitten for the first two to three critical months of its life. However, during this time, these maternal antibodies can block the young pet's response to vaccination. As they gradually fade away over those two to three months, there comes a point when vaccination may be initiated.. This point varies among puppies/kittens due to the varying amounts of maternal antibodies each receives. That's why puppy/kitten vaccination programs typically involve a series of shots given a few weeks apart.

Declining Immunity:

Without occasional exposure to the infectious agent in the environment, immunity to a specific organism decreases over time. This decline is more pronounced in older pets, and eventually, the immunity may become insufficient to prevent the disease. Natural exposure, known as asymptomatic boosting, helps to maintain effective immunity (Williams et al., n.d.-b).

Immune Suppression:

Some infections and certain medications, like anti-cancer drugs, can weaken the immune system. Even a properly vaccinated pet might become vulnerable to infection and disease if exposed to any viruses in the wild, as their immune was unable to mount a proper response to the vaccination. (Williams et al., n.d.-a).

New Strains of Organisms:

Infectious agents can have different strains or evolve into new ones that the vaccines may not directly cover. While the vaccine might provide some level of cross-protection or partial defense, it may not offer complete protection in these cases (Williams et al., n.d.-a).

Traditional veterinarians claim that for vaccines to work best, it's crucial to administer them when your pet is healthy and relaxed. If your dog or cat is already sick, a vaccine won't be effective in getting rid of the illness. Vaccines operate by triggering the immune system to identify and combat specific microorganisms like viruses or bacteria. Once vaccinated, the immune system is prepared to respond to future infections from those microorganisms. Essentially, vaccines attempt to simulate a real infection, enabling the immune system to mount an appropriate response.

What Are Antibody Titers, and Can They Replace Vaccinations?

Antibody titers are blood tests that measure specific antibodies in your pet's blood. While they don't replace vaccination programs, these tests help your veterinarian assess your pet's current protection against diseases.

Based on the results of these tests, veterinarians can customize your pet's vaccination schedule (AVMA, n.d.).

Why Do Young Pets Get Frequent Vaccinations?

Young animals, like puppies and kittens, are especially vulnerable to infections due to their immature immune systems. Although they get some immunity from their mother's milk, it's not long-lasting.

For the best defense during their early months, traditional veterinarians usually recommend a series of vaccinations, typically two to four weeks apart. Most puppies and kittens receive their final shot around four months of age, but your veterinarian might adjust this schedule based on your pet's unique circumstances and needs.

How Risky Is Pet Vaccination?

No vaccine is entirely risk-free or foolproof; the effectiveness of vaccines involves weighing potential risks against benefits.

Risks of Vaccination (Williams et al., n.d.-a):

- **Known side effects**: Occasional occurrences such as injection site-associated *feline fibrosarcoma*, (FISS) which is a cancerous tumor that originates in the connective fibrous tissue found at the ends of bones of the arm or legs. This often must be removed surgically.

- **Hypersensitivities**: Including anaphylaxis and common transient systemic effects like fever, lethargy, and loss of appetite.

- **Localized reactions**: Occurring at the injection site.

- **Immune homeostasis alterations**: Vaccines contribute to conditions like allergies or autoimmune diseases.

- **Post-vaccinal polyneuropathy**: Comparable to Guillain-Barre syndrome in humans, identified as coonhound paralysis in dogs.

In conclusion, the veterinarian's task of selecting vaccine products and designing vaccination programs is an intricate and challenging aspect of medical decision-making. It is crucial to recognize that vaccine products differ in both efficacy and safety, and their application is not universally indicated for all pets. While vaccination claims to protect a population of animals through the concept of herd immunity, it is essential to understand that not every individually vaccinated pet may be fully safeguarded. A profound knowledge of immunology, vaccinology, and the pathobiology of infectious diseases is imperative for the successful implementation of an effective vaccination program.

The overarching goal should be to formulate vaccination recommendations that balance the maintenance of clinically relevant immunity with the minimization of potential adverse events, ensuring the overall well-being of the animal population.

Chapter 3:

The Hidden Dangers of Vaccinating Pets

Veterinarians and scientists consistently advocate for vaccines as crucial in eliminating diseases in animals. However, they may overlook a significant aspect: While vaccines have been successful in reducing severe diseases, they can also lead to the emergence of persistent, hard-to-treat chronic conditions.

Vaccines can be a major challenge to the body's immune system by injecting weakened or killed organisms directly into the bloodstream, bypassing the body's natural defenses. This can result in immune system irregularities, causing chronic diseases in animals. Despite protecting against specific acute diseases, vaccines can weaken the immune system and bring underlying tendencies to the forefront, leading to issues like epilepsy, skin allergies, respiratory infections, and cancer. The current generation of animals may be experiencing the consequences of over-vaccination, suffering from the long-term effects of this medical practice (Loops, n.d.).

In this chapter, we will present major concerns regarding the dangers of vaccination, which include a debate on over-vaccination, adverse reactions to vaccines, immune-mediated diseases, sarcoma in cats, vaccinosis, and the harmful effects of adjuvants.

Over-Vaccination in Pets

Many pet owners are worried about over-vaccination. Some holistic veterinarians argue that vaccines for diseases like distemper and canine parvovirus can provide lifetime immunity after being given to adult animals, and do not need annual boosters. (Loops, n.d.).

Modified live virus vaccines, such as those for canine parvovirus, canine distemper, feline panleukopenia, calicivirus, and rhinotracheitis, require the virus in the vaccine to replicate and stimulate the immune system. However, in previously immunized pets, antibodies from the previous vaccine can block the replication of the new vaccinal virus. For example, after the second rabies vaccination, giving another rabies vaccine every one or two years doesn't improve the pets immune status.

Veterinarians are unsure about the right interval for vaccine re-administration to significantly enhance the immunity of a large portion of the pet population, but it's definitely not every one or two years (Loops, n.d.).

The practice of recommending annual re-vaccination began officially in 1978 without scientific proof of the need for such frequent booster shots. Good levels of humoral antibodies block the response to vaccine boosters, similar to how maternal antibodies block responses in some young animals. Administering

40

unnecessary vaccines provides no benefit and may even pose serious risks to the patient (The Science Has Been Done, 2003).

There are no scientific studies proving the need for cats or dogs to be re-vaccinated annually. Vaccinating for diseases caused by CDV, CPV2, FPLP, and FeLV every year doesn't show a different level of immunity compared to animals vaccinated early in life and challenged later on. Many veterinarians now acknowledge that annual re-vaccination with vaccines providing long-term immunity doesn't offer any measurable benefit. In almost all cases, there's no immunologic requirement for annual re-vaccination (The Science Has Been Done, 2003).

Adverse Health Effects Linked to Pet Vaccines

Unfortunately, a lot of traditional veterinarians are still not well-informed about how re-vaccination can lead to negative reactions in pets. Because of this, they continue to push for automatic re-vaccination instead of using antibody titer tests to check if their patients really need repeated annual shots against the same disease.

What's even more concerning is that many veterinarians stick to the same vaccine plans even when their patients have reacted badly to previous vaccines or have been diagnosed with health issues. They downplay the possibility of adverse vaccine events, even though adverse reactions are quite common, and there's a step up from mild to allergic reactions that can be life-threatening (The Science Has Been Done, 2003).

They also tend to overlook the potential long-term effects of vaccines. For instance, vaccine-related sarcomas in cats can occur anywhere between 2 months to 10 years after vaccination.

The first set of vaccine adverse reactions mentioned by the AVMA usually show up within hours after vaccination:

- discomfort and swelling at the vaccination site

- mild fever

- reduced appetite and activity

- sneezing, mild coughing, or respiratory signs two to five days after intranasal vaccines

The AVMA says it's common for pets to experience some or all of these reactions. If they last for more than a few days and cause significant discomfort, it's important to contact your veterinarian.

The second, more serious group of reactions can occur within minutes to hours after vaccination:

- persistent vomiting or diarrhea

- itchy, bumpy skin ("hives")

- swelling around the face, neck, or eyes

- severe coughing or difficulty breathing

- collapse

The AVMA stresses that these reactions can be life-threatening and are medical emergencies. Immediate veterinary care is crucial if any of these signs develop (*The Science Has Been Done*, 2003).

The AVMA describes a feline injection-site sarcoma (FISS) as a "small, firm swelling under the skin" that should start to disappear within a couple of weeks. However, if it persists for more than three weeks or seems to be getting larger, it's advised to contact the veterinarian. The truth of the matter (which AVMA conveniently fails to mention) is that these are malignant tumors that come back no matter how many times they are surgically removed. This often leads to the need to amputate the affected limb. (*The Science Has Been Done*, 2003).

Adjuvants Used in Vaccines and the Dangers Associated with Them

Vaccine adjuvants are substances that boost the immune response to vaccine antigens, which are the components that stimulate the immune system. In the early 20th century, a French veterinarian named Gaston Ramon found that adding various substances like calcium chloride, saponins, starch, vegetable oil, and bacteria to the "anatoxine diphtérique" vaccine for horses increased inflammation at the injection site (Burakova et al., 2018). This enhanced the production of antibodies against toxins. Since then, adjuvants have played a crucial role in vaccine technology for both animals and humans. In essence, they drastically increase the amount of inflammation that occurs after vaccination, which is believed to lead to a more robust immune response.

They activate the cells that present antigens and release them slowly to keep the immune stimulation going. So far, many substances from organic, inorganic, synthetic, and natural sources have shown the ability to boost immune responses and act as strong adjuvants. Creating effective vaccines that use purified parts or inactive microbes needs reliable adjuvants, or they don't work well. This is important because the antigens in these vaccines are often not as good at triggering the immune system as modified live microbes (Burakova et al., 2018).

However, adjuvants come with risks as they can cause local reactions, including inflammation and granulomas or sterile abscesses. In dogs, rabies or distemper combination vaccines are most often associated with local reactions, while in cats, rabies vaccines are most frequently linked to local non-neoplastic reactions. (Burakova et al, 2018).

Finding the right adjuvant is crucial, and cost-effectiveness is a big consideration. Developing vaccines for animals is different from making vaccines for humans. In humans, the individual's health is the top priority, but for animals, controlling diseases has to be cost-effective. Human vaccines can be quite expensive, often over $100 per dose, while animal vaccines are usually priced lower. This results in limited funding for researching and developing animal vaccines compared to human vaccines, impacting the available choices and, consequently, the quality of adjuvants for use (Burakova et al., 2018).

Additionally, developing vaccines for animals has less stringent regulations and fewer rules to follow compared to human vaccines. Some compounds that can't be used in human vaccines due to safety concerns are allowed in animal vaccines, resulting in more adverse health effects to the pets. Recently, there's been a growing interest in reducing side effects from vaccines and creating specific types of immunity, leading to the development of many new adjuvants. (Burakova et al, 2018).

Suffice it to say that choosing or creating adjuvants for animal vaccines requires considering several important factors. These include how well they work in the specific animal, their ability to quickly and effectively build lasting immunity, ensuring they're safe for animals, following food safety rules, being practical for large-scale production, and, importantly, being cost-effective.

Figuring out the right adjuvant or combination that meets all these criteria is a big challenge in developing vaccines for animals.

Immune-Mediated Diseases

Sometimes, tricking the immune system with a vaccine can backfire, causing the body to start attacking the body's own cells, leading to what is known as immune-mediated diseases. In animals, the most common ones involve the immune system mistakenly destroying important cells like red blood cells or platelets. Instead of fighting off harmful invaders, the body creates inflammation that targets its own tissues (Purdue University, n.d.).

This can cause serious problems like anemia, heart rhythm issues, and clotting disorders. These are some of the known adverse effects of pet vaccines.

Treatment of immune mediated diseases often involves medications to suppress the immune system, aiming to reduce or eliminate the inappropriate response. In many cases, dogs and cats might need immune-suppressive therapy for about four to six months. In severe cases, this treatment could continue for the rest of their lives.

However, while these medications help treat the disease, they also bring risks. Suppressing the immune system makes animals more susceptible to other infections like skin or urinary tract infections.

Sarcomas/Cancers Linked to Vaccines/Adjuvants (FISS)

Sarcomas are harmful tumors that can show up weeks, months, or even years after a vaccination is administered to a cat. Feline injection-site sarcomas (FISS), also known as vaccine-associated sarcomas (VAS), often happens due to the feline rabies vaccine and the feline leukemia virus (FeLV) vaccine (*Preventative Medicine*, 2013).

These tumors are aggressive and can spread to nearby tissues and even other parts of the body, making the outlook not very hopeful. The time it takes for a sarcoma to develop after a vaccine can vary a lot, from 2 months to 10 years (*Preventative Medicine*, 2013).

Veterinarians have known for a long time that vaccines cause sarcomas in cats. In 1991, three years after Pennsylvania made rabies vaccinations mandatory for cats, experts at the University of Pennsylvania found a causal link between increased sarcomas and cat vaccinations. Soon after, the University of California at Davis connected FeLV vaccines to sarcomas (*Preventative Medicine*, 2013).

Most of the first sarcomas found in cats were between the shoulder blades because that's where vaccines were usually given before the mid-1990s. It's believed that the process of injecting vaccines might cause chronic inflammation, leading to sarcoma formation. The role of adjuvants (like those with aluminum) and local inflammation in causing FISS is not entirely clear. Recent studies suggest that vaccines and other injections could be risk factors for FISS. Some cats may not control inflammation well, which might explain how it turns into a sarcoma (*Preventative Medicine*, 2013).

In 1996, a group called the Vaccine-Associated Feline Sarcoma Task Force wanted to figure out which vaccines were causing sarcomas in cats. They told vets to give rabies vaccines in the right rear leg and FeLV vaccines in the left rear leg. The shots had to be low on the legs, far from the body, so if needed, part of the leg could be amputated as a cancer treatment (AVMA, n.d.).

After these new recommendations, there were fewer sarcomas in the neck area for the next 10 years. However, there were more sarcomas in the legs and belly, especially on the right side (AVMA, n.d.).

Because most sarcomas were now in the right rear legs, it seemed like the rabies vaccine was the main cause of cancer. The importance of injecting low on the leg became clear when more sarcomas appeared on the side of the belly after 1996. If a cat is crouched, injecting in what seems like the leg can end up being in the side of the belly when the cat stands up (AVMA, n.d.).

In 2013, a team of vet researchers suggested that giving vaccines in the tail could make treating sarcomas easier and less disfiguring. This might encourage more cat owners to get cancer treatment for their pets. A sad reality is that no matter how many times you remove it surgically, the sarcoma tends to grow back, and limb amputation is almost always required to save the animal. (AVMA, n.d.).

Integrative Veterinarians who look at the big picture focus on giving animals the vaccines they really need, considering their immunity, age, lifestyle, and actual exposure to risks (*Preventative Medicine*, 2013).

Not many veterinarians think about the real risks of indoor pets catching infections from other animals. Most diseases in cats spread when outdoor cats interact with infected ones.

But what about indoor cats who only step out for walks once or twice a day? Their risk is almost zero. The danger is in giving too many vaccines to these well-protected pets who don't face many risks. In these cases, there is all risk, and virtually no benefit to vaccinating.

The Problem of Vaccinosis

Vaccinosis is a long term, steady decline in the pets health due to a buildup of adjuvants, foreign protein, and preservatives from vaccines, that the body has no way of eliminating.

When pets have reactions to vaccines, like feeling tired or having flu-like symptoms, it's something regular veterinarians agree happens occasionally. Even severe reactions, like anaphylactic shock, are seen as rare problems as a result of vaccination.

But there's another issue called vaccinosis. Only holistic and integrative vets talk about it, although some regular veterinarians are starting to consider it more. This happens when a pets immune system reacts to the vaccines, but there wasn't any obvious immediate problem after the shot. It's not just a response to the virus in the vaccine but also to the chemicals, adjuvants, and preservatives in the vaccine, including possible genetic changes. This has become more recognized, especially with the ongoing potential side effects of COVID-19 vaccines acknowledged by health organizations (Becker, 2023a).

Dr. Richard Pitcairn, who is an expert in veterinary homeopathy, defines vaccinosis as a prolonged disturbance caused by vaccines. It leads to mental, emotional, and physical changes, sometimes becoming a permanent condition (Becker, 2023a).

According to Dr. Pitcairn, vaccines meant to protect pets from diseases can create ongoing problems that mimic the diseases they were supposed to prevent. This happens when natural viruses are changed in a lab to make vaccines. While the natural virus would trigger a strong immune response, the modified lab virus in the vaccine doesn't provoke much of a reaction from the animal's immune system. Instead of helping to mount an immune response, the adjuvants and preservatives used in the vaccine can cause lasting changes in the animal's body that may lead to other diseases, such as immune mediated diseases. (Becker, 2023a).

Vaccines are quite different from natural diseases in how they work in an animal's body. They contain a concoction of irritants such as heavy metals, modified bacteria/cell cultures, adjuvants, foreign proteins, and chemical preservatives.

These toxins are injected directly into the muscle, blood and lymph, skipping the usual defense lines like the skin, nose, and saliva. So, not only is the modified virus in the vaccine unnatural, but the way it gets into an animal's body is also not normal. When you consider this unnatural route of administration, it's easier to understand that vaccines can, and often do, cause abnormal immune reactions.

Symptoms of Vaccinosis

Common symptoms include (Becker, 2023a):

- feeling tired
- losing hair
- change in fur color where the shot was given
- fever
- soreness
- stiffness
- not wanting to eat
- eye infection (conjunctivitis)
- sneezing
- sores in the mouth

More serious symptoms may include (Becker, 2023a):

- weakened immune system
- changes in behavior

- a skin condition called vitiligo

- losing weight

- less milk production in females

- trouble walking (lameness)

- lumps and pockets of infection (granulomas and abscesses)

- red, itchy welts (hives)

- swelling of the face

- extreme allergic reaction

- breathing problems

- eye inflammation due to allergies

- severe conditions like cancer at the injection site

- life-threatening allergic reaction (anaphylaxis)

- immune system attacking joints (autoimmune arthritis)

- joint inflammation (polyarthritis)

- bone disease (hypertrophic osteodystrophy)

- immune system destroying red blood cells (autoimmune hemolytic anemia)

- low platelet count due to immune system attack (immune-mediated thrombocytopenia)

- thyroid inflammation (thyroiditis)

- kidney inflammation (glomerulonephritis)

- heart inflammation (myocarditis)

- brain or nerve inflammation (encephalitis or

polyneuritis)

- seizures

- loss of pregnancy (abortion)

- birth defects in newborns

- death of unborn babies (embryotic or fetal death)

- trouble having babies (infertility)

The severe nature of the symptoms of vaccinosis underscores the need to administer vaccines when they are absolutely necessary, or legally mandated. The immunity from vaccines can last for many years or even the animal's whole life. However, getting more vaccines may not work well because existing antibodies can interfere. Still, the common practice in veterinary guidelines is to focus on how many vaccines can be given and how often, usually annually, even though its safety and effectiveness is questionable (Becker, 2023a).

Many integrative and holistic veterinarians suggest a safer and more humane approach to vaccinations. The idea is to give only the necessary vaccines needed to protect pets from diseases they might actually encounter. Here are some examples (Becker, 2022):

If your cat stays indoors all the time, you might want to think about the risks of all the recommended vaccinations. If they never go outside and have almost zero chance of catching dangerous diseases, you might decide to skip vaccines.

Generally, if you're a careful pet parent and your cat lives indoors without meeting other cats, their risk of getting sick from diseases is almost zero. Some experts believe giving too many vaccines is a big reason why the health of house cats is declining (Becker, 2022). If your indoor cat doesn't interact with other cats, their risk is pretty much nonexistent.

If your pet does have a chance of getting sick, it's a good idea to find an integrative veterinarian. These non-traditional vets focus on proactive health care and are usually more cautious about giving too many vaccines. They might also know about ways to help your pet detox from vaccines, which regular veterinarians might not be aware of.

You can ask for a vaccine titer test to check your pet's immunity against diseases they were vaccinated for in their first year (kitten/puppy shots). If they're already immune, there's no need for more vaccines. Don't keep vaccinating your pet if they are already protected (Becker, 2022).

If your pet needs a booster shot or a vaccine they haven't had before, consider the following (Becker, 2023a):

- The vaccine is for a serious disease that could be deadly and is common in your area.

- Your pet could be exposed to the disease.

- The vaccine is recognized for its safety and efficacy.

If your pet does need a vaccine, ask your veterinarian for Thuja, a homeopathic remedy that can help counteract the harmful effects of vaccines, excluding rabies vaccines.

Rabies vaccines are required by law in many places. Holistic veterinarians suggest using the one-year non-adjuvanted vaccine for pets and an extra dose of the homeopathic rabies vaccine detoxifier, Lyssin. If your pet is a kitten, it's better to give the rabies vaccine after four months of age, preferably closer to six months, to lower the risk of an adverse reaction (Becker, 2023a).

Don't give your pet a vaccine if they have had a bad reaction to one before.

The main goal of vaccination is to make sure pets are protected. Giving a bunch of vaccines doesn't help if the dog or cat's immune system doesn't respond well. It's like getting all the bad stuff from the vaccines without any of the good. This way, the whole process appears counterproductive as the only reason a pet is put through the pain and stress of vaccination is to give immunity against dangerous diseases—so if that result is missing, what's the point of the whole exercise?

To conclude, it is fair to say that the main takeaway to consider before vaccinating is the risk of exposure. If your cats stay inside all the time, or if your dogs are always on a leash or in a fenced area when outside, there's not much risk. Other things to consider are if the disease is so serious that getting vaccinated is necessary. It's important to know that vaccines can have risks. Only vaccinate if there's a real threat.

Chapter 4:

The Rabies Vaccine—A

Different Approach

Rabies is a viral disease that affects the nervous system of mammals, including humans, dogs, cats, and foxes. The virus is mainly found in the saliva and brain of infected animals, particularly dogs, and is usually transmitted through bites. Bats also play a significant role in certain regions. When there's a high presence of the virus in wildlife, it increases the chances of transmission to domestic animals and humans (O'Niell, n.d.).

Being a disease that can pass between animals and humans, rabies is considered zoonotic. The incubation period varies, but once symptoms appear, it is almost always fatal, with a 99% chance of domestic dogs transmitting the virus to humans. However, both domestic and wild animals can be affected. Rabies spreads through saliva, typically through bites, scratches, or direct contact with mucous membranes (like eyes, mouth, or open wounds) (O'Niell, n.d.).

Rabies can be transmitted by various wild carnivore host species like bats, foxes, raccoons, skunks, jackals, and mongooses, causing infections in humans and pets. However, bites from rodents are not known to transmit rabies.

Children between 5 and 14 years old are frequent victims. While bites are the primary mode of transmission, scratches and licks can also lead to infection, though less commonly. Under certain conditions, inhalation of highly concentrated viral particles may also cause transmission. The virus gains access to the nervous system through direct inoculation into peripheral nerves or infection of surrounding tissue, such as muscle cells, with subsequent nerve entry at the neuromuscular junction (O'Niell, n.d.).

History of the Disease and Development of Vaccines

For ages, rabies has been a terrifying threat, with its deadly consequences evident once someone was bitten by an infected animal. The term "rabies" could possibly trace its origins to the Sanskrit term "rabhas," signifying violence, or the Latin term "*rabere*," denoting a state of rage. The ancient Greeks referred to rabies as "*lyssa*," signifying violence. Today, the virus responsible for rabies falls under the genus Lyssa Virus. (O'Niell, n.d.).

In ancient India, around 3000 B.C., the god of death was symbolized by a dog as its messenger. The first recorded instance of rabies causing death in both dogs and humans dates back to 2300 B.C. in the Mosaic Esmuna Code of Babylon. Babylonians had to pay a penalty if their dog passed on rabies to another individual (O'Niell, n.d.).

Moving ahead to the first century A.D., the Roman scholar Celsus correctly identified that rabies spreads through the saliva of the biting animal. However, he proposed an incorrect cure, suggesting holding the victim underwater. Unfortunately, those who didn't drown ultimately succumbed to rabies.

The first effective treatment for rabies emerged in the 1880s when a French chemistry teacher named Louis Pasteur was experimenting with chicken cholera. While working with virulent cultures, he observed that exposure to the elements made them no longer disease-causing. He also found that chickens given this weakened or "attenuated strain" became immune to fresh, virulent cultures. Pasteur successfully used an attenuated vaccine against anthrax in cattle, leading him to focus on rabies (O'Niell, n.d.).

Though his initial animal studies were promising, Pasteur wanted to refine his vaccine before trying it on humans. On July 6, 1885, he treated a boy attacked by rabid dogs with 13 inoculations in 11 days, and the boy made a full recovery (O'Niell, n.d.). Since then, thousands of people have received his post-exposure prophylactic vaccine.

Some people still underestimate the need for rabies vaccinations in cats. Wild animal rabies, mainly involving raccoons, skunks, foxes, and bats, poses a risk. Bats are particularly dangerous as rabid bats can go unnoticed and easily enter narrow spaces, exposing both humans and pets day and night (O'Niell, n.d.).

Louis Pasteur's development of the first rabies vaccine in 1885 significantly reduced the prevalence of this deadly disease in human and domestic animal populations in developed countries through widespread vaccination.

The Real Issue With Modern-Day Rabies Vaccine

A major concern with current vaccines, especially rabies vaccines, is that most of them contain adjuvants like mercury or aluminum. These elements are highly toxic and are not well-tolerated by vaccine recipients in many cases. It's crucial to replace these adjuvants in rabies vaccines (Becker & Schultz, 2014).

The amount of rabies vaccine given is also a topic of debate among veterinarians. State laws mandate a one-milliliter dose for all dogs, regardless of size. Many integrative veterinarians believe that a one-size-fits-all approach puts smaller dogs at a higher risk of vaccine reactions, (Becker & Schultz, 2014).

Another issue is the unnecessary over-vaccination due to state mandates. Certain viruses, like feline panleukopenia, canine distemper, canine hepatitis, and canine parvovirus, create long-lasting immune memory cells. This means once an animal has immune memory and circulating antibodies, they cannot be reinfected. While they may still carry the virus in their urine or stool, they cannot be reinfected themselves (Schultz, 2016).

While some vaccines provide lasting protection, rabies vaccines don't offer sterile immunity. Even though rabies vaccinations need to be repeated, they might not need to be as frequent as they currently are. Many pet owners wonder why there are only one-year and three-year rabies vaccines and not, for example, seven or twelve-year vaccines. Dr. Schultz, a top Veterinarian with over 40 years of experience in treating various animals, is currently conducting studies to prove that rabies immunity can last for at least seven years. If successful, this research could allow us to extend the time between re-vaccinations. However, such studies are expensive and time-consuming, which is why, until now, no one has undertaken research to prove that we can go beyond the three-year mark (Becker, 2018).

Alarming Study Findings on Protective Level of Rabies Antibodies in Vaccinated Dogs

A study in Chennai, India, looking into the effectiveness of rabies vaccinations in dogs uncovered concerning findings. Out of 180 young and adult dogs, 60% (108) didn't have enough antibodies to provide protection within a year of their last rabies vaccination despite having a history of previous vaccinations. This high percentage of dogs not responding to the vaccine raises concerns about how vaccines are administered, distributed, stored, and managed for quality and potency in India. Further studies are necessary to determine if these results are specific to a certain region or if similar non-responsive cases exist in other areas as well (Yale et al., 2021).

Revisiting Rabies Vaccine Schedule: Examining Legal Requirements

Rabies vaccines are required by law in all 50 states because rabies is a deadly and zoonotic disease. Like all vaccines, rabies shots can cause reactions ranging from mild to severe, including anaphylaxis and death. Some states allow for medical exemptions from rabies vaccines for pets who are ill or have had an adverse reaction in the past (Schultz, 2016).

The good news is that all states now have a three-year re-vaccination plan after the second vaccine. However, some county and city laws may differ, so it's crucial to check with your local animal control for details. There's a push to change the recommendation so that animals vaccinated for rabies between 12 to 24 weeks old don't need re-vaccination every three years (Becker & Schultz, 2014).

Every U.S. state now has a three-year rabies law, but city laws may be more restrictive, requiring yearly or bi-yearly rabies vaccines. Holistic veterinarians remind pet owners that they have the power to change laws if their location requires more frequent vaccinations. Scientifically, there's no need to vaccinate animals more often than every three years, as all major vaccine manufacturers have conducted minimum three-year studies showing their products provide at least three years of immunity (Becker & Schultz, 2014). This should assure veterinarians and pet owners that it's safe to go three years between vaccinations, regardless of the product used.

Re-vaccinating your animal more often won't improve herd immunity or protect them better against rabies. Those who don't vaccinate their pets will likely continue to avoid it, so the need for more frequent rabies vaccines seems like a punishment for responsible pet owners who follow the law. Dr. Schultz, with 40 years of experience, points out that most one- and three-year rabies vaccines are similar. However, there's a one-year feline rabies vaccine without adjuvants, but there isn't a corresponding three-year version yet (Becker & Schultz, 2014).

Dr. Schultz explains that the adjuvant-free one-year feline rabies vaccine is new technology, acting like a modified live vaccine without live rabies. The cat's immune system sees this vaccine as live. Studies by the developing company showed 100% protection against rabies even after three years. However, the USDA didn't issue a three-year license because there weren't enough deaths in the control (non-vaccinated) group of cats. Even in a second round of studies with fewer non-vaccinated cat deaths, the USDA still refused to issue a one-year license for the product (Becker & Schultz, 2014).

When it comes to vaccine-associated sarcoma (VAS) in cats, Dr. Schultz suggests opting for the non-adjuvanted one-year rabies vaccine rather than the three-year vaccine with adjuvants. The non-adjuvanted one-year vaccine doesn't trigger an inflammatory response at the injection site (a sign of tumor development), unlike adjuvanted rabies vaccines, which are known to increase VAS. Even for genetically predisposed cats, it's assumed that the non-adjuvanted product, even given yearly, is less harmful than the adjuvanted vaccine (Schultz, 2016).

Since cats are more prone to developing sarcoma, the trend in feline vaccines is moving toward non-adjuvanted products. Adjuvanted products are more likely to cause adverse reactions in general across all species. The future goal in vaccine development is to have fewer adjuvanted vaccines and to create new adjuvants that are less likely to cause adverse reactions (Schultz, 2016).

The recommended rabies protocol suggests the first vaccine after four months of age, a re-vaccination in a year, followed by another in three years, and then every three years. Dr. Schultz emphasizes that this protocol is due to the law, not because a three-year interval is necessary for immunity. The law doesn't consider if an animal already has immunity from a prior vaccine; it mandates vaccinations every one, two, or three years (Schultz, 2016).

If you choose not to re-vaccinate your pet for rabies, it's your decision, but it's essential to know it goes against the law. If Dr. Schultz's seven-year rabies study proves the vaccine is effective for that duration, it could lead to a change in vaccination laws, potentially reducing the number of rabies vaccines a dog receives in its lifetime to just two.

Most Common Mistakes Made With the Rabies Vaccine

In the United States, many places mandate adult pets to be re-vaccinated every year or three years, regardless of their antibody status. This approach is scientifically flawed because the primary goal of vaccination should be to safely protect pets from disease, not just to meet administrative requirements or deadlines (Becker, 2018).

Some veterinarians make the mistake of vaccinating young pets earlier than necessary. Pet owners should wait until their pet reaches the oldest age allowed by law before giving the first rabies vaccination. This age varies by state, with some allowing it at six months and others even earlier. Giving the rabies vaccine too early can lead to various problems, as studies indicate, including a higher chance of vaccine failure, especially in puppies under three months old (Becker & Schultz, 2014).

Another common error made by some veterinarians is advocating for more frequent vaccinations. Holistic veterinarians strongly advise pet owners to request the three-year vaccine after the second rabies shot for the rest of their pet's life. The three-year vaccine provides the same protection required by law as the one-year vaccine but at less frequent intervals. This results in fewer vaccines over your pet's lifetime and reduces the risk of adverse reactions (Becker, 2018).

Some veterinarians also administer a combination vaccine for other diseases alongside the rabies vaccine.

However, experts emphasize that rabies vaccinations should never be given simultaneously with or at the same time as another vaccine. They should be administered alone, with a gap of at least two weeks from all other vaccinations. (Becker, 2018).

Pet owners are advised to opt for titer tests for other diseases, and hopefully, with potential changes in laws, rabies titers may also be accepted as proof of protective immunity. This can prevent unnecessary over-vaccination and help identify animals with vaccine failure (Becker, 2018).

To alleviate the strain on a pet's body caused by the vaccine, holistic veterinarians recommend a homeopathic detox remedy for the rabies vaccine called **lyssin,** especially if the pet has experienced an adverse reaction. It's important to observe the injection site closely after each vaccination. If there is any inflammation, abnormality, or change in the appearance of the skin, such as a lump, irritation, or heat, it's crucial to contact a veterinarian immediately (Becker, 2018).

Study Validating Rabies Vaccine Protection Lasts Five Years

A recent study supported by The Rabies Challenge Fund indicates that the rabies vaccine remains effective for at least five years and doesn't have to be given annually. The Rabies Challenge Fund, led by Kris Christine, immunologist Dr. Ronald Schultz, and Dr. Dodds, conducted the study in collaboration with the University of Wisconsin at a privately owned veterinary Beagle breeding facility. Beagles, the average size for dog vaccine testing, received two doses of the rabies vaccine (Becker, 2021).

In the planned five-year and seven-year studies, at least 20 dogs were to be challenged with rabies virus to demonstrate their protection from vaccination, while others would serve as controls. When the dogs were challenged after six and a half years of vaccination, it was found that 80% of them survived, meeting USDA standards. So, conservatively, we can say that at five years, without a doubt, 80% of the challenged animals in the study survived. The unvaccinated animals that were challenged were humanely euthanized (Becker, 2021).

After completing the five-year challenge study, Dr. Dodds and her colleagues considered asking the USDA to extend the licensing to five years for the rabies vaccine. However, due to opposition from other vaccine manufacturers and the USDA's existing workload, Dr. Dodds decided to wait (Becker, 2021).

Dr. John Robb, another eminent veterinarian, is actively raising awareness about this issue on a national level. The scientists involved in the study are optimistic that this increased awareness will encourage changes in this requirement, potentially influencing states one by one (Becker, 2021).

In conclusion, while the rabies vaccine remains a crucial and legally mandated aspect of pet care, recent studies suggest that a reevaluation of its dosage and frequency may be warranted. The potential toxicity of adjuvants in the vaccine raises concerns, and advocates are advocating for their replacement with less harmful alternatives. It becomes imperative for the scientific community to invest in further research aimed at developing more effective, less repetitive, and minimally adverse effect-inducing rabies vaccines. By continuously reassessing and improving our approach to rabies vaccination, we can ensure the health and well-being of our pets while aligning with the evolving landscape of veterinary science and understanding.

Chapter 5

How Pet Vaccines Are Licensed and Regulated

More and more people in the U.S. are becoming pet owners. A recent survey discovered that 67% of households across the country have at least one pet (Fox, n.d.). This has increased emphasis on issues related to pet health in general and preventing diseases in particular.

As explained by the Center for Veterinary Biologics–Licensing and Policy Development (CVB-LPD) guidelines, vaccine production begins with research and development (R&D) activities, which include preclinical studies to demonstrate the quality, safety, and efficacy of the products. These studies follow international reference standards such as good laboratory practice (GLP) for preclinical studies and good clinical practice (GCP) for clinical studies (AAHA, 2022b).

Before a vaccine can be used in a country, it must receive regulatory approval from the competent authority. This involves submitting a dossier detailing the starting materials, manufacturing processes, in-process controls, and finished product controls. The dossier also includes tests conducted to demonstrate the quality, safety, and efficacy of the vaccine. Regulatory approval ensures compliance with local product regulatory requirements before the vaccine can be released for use (AAHA, 2022b).

Once the competent authority approves the vaccine, it can be produced in a manufacturing facility authorized by them. This facility must meet national requirements and have the necessary equipment, facilities, and staff for production and quality control. The manufacturing site is regularly inspected by experienced official inspectors to ensure compliance (AAHA, 2022b).

Quality assurance is essential in making sure that vaccines are pure, safe, and effective throughout the production process.

In this chapter, we'll look closely at how pet vaccines are licensed, including the roles of regulatory authorities. We'll explore the scientific evidence used to assess vaccine effectiveness during the licensing process. Lastly, we'll discuss how conflicts of interest, such as funding from big pharmaceutical companies to academic and research institutions, can influence the quality of scientific research aimed at improving pet vaccines.

How Pet Vaccine Licensure Works

The U.S. Department of Agriculture (USDA) oversees and requires the licensing of biologics under the Virus-Serum-Toxin Act. This law ensures that veterinary biologics, like (pet) vaccines, are safe, effective, and free from contaminants. The USDA's Animal and Plant Health Inspection Service provides manufacturers with detailed guidelines to follow, and they inspect manufacturing facilities before granting a license. These inspections continue periodically to ensure ongoing compliance (AAHA, 2022b).

Manufacturers must meet strict standards not only for their facilities but also for the materials they use, such as seed viruses and cell lines. Once a vaccine is licensed, manufacturers are not allowed to make significant changes to their manufacturing process to maintain product consistency (AAHA, 2022b).

Different types of licenses are issued for vaccines based on their specific categories.

Fully licensed products meet strict requirements to ensure they are pure, safe, potent, and effective. Conditional licenses, on the other hand, are issued quickly in emergencies or special circumstances where there's a limited market or local situation. These products must still meet safety and efficacy standards. Imported products are allowed for distribution and sale if they meet the same standards as fully licensed ones. This usually happens when there aren't enough USDA-licensed products available, and there's a real risk of new animal diseases emerging (AAHA, 2022b).

Along with these, the licensing submission must show that the product can be made and used without harming animal or human health, food safety, or the environment (AAHA, 2022b).

What Regulatory Bodies Exist (USA Market) and Their Role

All vaccines for animals sold in the U.S., including those for diseases like pseudorabies, must follow a law called the Virus Serum Toxin Act (VSTA), which started in 1913 but was updated in 1985 (*Veterinary Biologic*, n.d.).

This law says that most vaccines need a license to be sold, and a group called the Licensing and Policy Development unit in the Center for Veterinary Biologics (CVB), which is part of the Animal and Plant Health Inspection Service (APHIS) of the USDA, makes sure this happens. The law gives power to the USDA Secretary to make rules about how these vaccines are made and sold, both inside and outside the U.S. The VSTA also says that it's illegal to sell or transport bad or unsafe vaccines unless they are made in a place licensed by the USDA and follow their rules (*Veterinary Biologic*, n.d.).

Before bringing in any veterinary vaccines from outside the U.S., the USDA needs to give permission first. They also have the power to check these vaccines before they come in. If someone breaks the rules, the USDA can take away their license to make or sell these vaccines or even stop them from doing business altogether. They can also take away the vaccines or stop them from being sold (*Veterinary Biologic*, n.d.).

In the U.S., licenses for animal vaccines are given out by a part of the Department of Agriculture USDA, called the Animal Plant Health Inspection Service (APHIS), in a section called Veterinary Services (VS), specifically in the Center for Veterinary Biologics (CVB). The VST Act, which controls these licenses, is looked after by APHIS within the USDA, especially in the Veterinary Services section of the CVB (*Veterinary Biologic*, n.d.).

Inside the CVB, there are three main teams that handle the licensing, checking, and testing of animal vaccines (*Veterinary Biologic*, n.d.):

1. The Center for Veterinary Biologics–Licensing and Policy Development (CVB-LPD) in Riverdale, Maryland, handles things before licenses are given out. This includes looking at applications for licenses and making rules and policies for the program.

2. The Center for Veterinary Biologics–Inspection and Compliance (CVB-IC) in Ames, Iowa, takes care of things after licenses are given. They inspect places where the vaccines are made, approve batches of vaccines for sale, handle complaints from customers, and check if anyone is breaking the rules.

3. The Center for Veterinary Biologics–Laboratory (CVB-L) in Ames, Iowa, does tests on the ingredients and batches of vaccines, both before and after they're licensed. They also work on making better ways to test these vaccines.

The Center for Veterinary Biologics–Laboratory (CVB-L) offers some extra tests called Supplemental Assay Methods (SAM). These tests help with checking if animal vaccines are safe and work well. Some of the tests include (*Veterinary Biologic*, n.d.):

- Tests that measure antibodies for pseudorabies using a certain method.

- Tests that check the strength of the pseudorabies virus.

- Tests that measure how well antibodies can fight pseudorabies.

When licensing live animal vaccines, especially those made with biotechnology, another law called the National Environmental Policy Act (NEPA) from 1969 needs to be taken into account before licensing. This law makes sure that when new vaccines are made, they don't harm the environment, especially if they're tested outside the U.S. (*Veterinary Biologic*, n.d.).

How Robust Is the Scientific Evidence for Licensing Pet Vaccines?

The USDA ensures that vaccines meet scientific standards before granting licenses. This involves reviewing the quality of clinical trials, the methods used in experiments, and how results are presented and interpreted. They consider different aspects (*Veterinary Biologic*, n.d.):

- **Type of study:** Studies can be clinical or nonclinical, experimental or observational, and exploratory or confirmatory. Exploratory studies aim to understand features of the material or process being studied, while confirmatory studies support final production or testing specifications.

- **Scientific standards:** Studies should be designed, conducted, analyzed, and reported using sound scientific principles. Manufacturers are advised to follow accepted standards for objectivity and scientific rigor in all studies and to show this in associated documents.

- **Statistical principles:** Manufacturers must ensure that statistical methods are applied correctly throughout the research process, from forming the initial question to presenting the final results.

- **Submission:** Manufacturers should send a study plan to the CVB for review at least 60 days before starting. If there are big problems with the plan, the CVB might ask for changes. Before starting a confirmatory study, manufacturers need CVB's agreement. But this doesn't mean they approve everything about how the study is done or what the results will be.

- **Sensitivity analysis:** When looking at statistical results, manufacturers must consider how bias might affect them. Bias can be hard to see, so it's important to check if the conclusions are still valid, even if there are problems with the data or how it's analyzed.

- **Study animals:** Manufacturers should use animals that are most likely to get sick from the disease, regardless of their age. These animals should also be able to catch the disease the vaccine is meant to prevent. The study plan should explain why certain animals of a specific age and sex are being used.

- **Observations:** Keep an eye on animals after giving them the vaccine, looking for signs that the vaccine could become harmful. People running the tests should watch out for any signs that the vaccine might be causing problems for the animals (*Veterinary Biologic*, n.d.).

Vaccine makers need to carry out specific tests on the vaccine before it can be approved for use. Some of these tests include (*Veterinary Biologic*, n.d.):

- **Virus identity test:** To check if the vaccine contains the right virus, samples from each batch of the vaccine are tested.

- **Target animal safety tests:** Early in the

development of the vaccine, its safety for the animals it's meant for should be shown. This includes checking if a single dose is safe, if giving too much is safe, and if repeated doses are safe.

- **Increase in virulence tests:** With live vaccines, there's a worry that the vaccine might become stronger and cause harm. These tests make sure the vaccine doesn't become more harmful with time.

- **Assessing risk to the environment:** Live vaccines can sometimes spread to other animals and stay in the environment. Before approval, it's important to see if this could happen and if it would be harmful.

- **Laboratory efficacy test:** The vaccine's effectiveness is checked using statistically reliable studies on the animals it's meant for. These studies should show how well the vaccine works in different situations described on the product label.

- **Interference tests:** Tests are done to see if different vaccines from the same maker or given to the same animal around the same time might interfere with each other. This ensures that the vaccines work as they should.

- **Batch/serial purity test:** Before the vaccine is released, a sample from each batch is tested to make sure it's pure, safe, and effective, following the maker's approved manufacturing process (*Veterinary Biologic*, n.d.).

Conflicts of Interest Compromising Research/Recommendations

Conflicts of interest can make vaccine safety research less reliable. The companies funding the research might have their own interests, which could affect how they study vaccine side effects. Vaccine makers, government health agencies, and medical journals might not want to admit that vaccines can be risky because of financial or bureaucratic reasons. If conflicts of interest in vaccine safety research are minimized, it could help make the research more fair and trustworthy and restore confidence in vaccination programs (Fox, n.d.).

Conflict of interest is not limited to big players; sometimes, veterinarians can also be susceptible to it. For example, veterinarians may be torn between making money by encouraging vaccinations, and putting the best interests of the animals first. This problem is similar to what's been happening in human medicine, which was recently questioned by the U.S. Institute of Medicine (Fox, n.d.).

These conflicts of interest can be found throughout the veterinary education system, where big drug and pet food companies have a lot of influence. This influence can be seen in how veterinarians practice every day.

One issue is unnecessary vaccinations. Many veterinarians give pets shots every year that they don't really need. The relationships between these companies and veterinarians are being questioned in human medicine, so it's worth asking if the same should happen in veterinary medicine. Are these corporate interests affecting the quality of care our pets receive?

Partnerships between the corporate sector and academia extend to various veterinary colleges, where companies may have chairs and professorships named after them due to their donations. The implications of such collaborations on issues like poor diets, over-medication, and hyperimmunization in companion animals are complex. There's a concern that vested interests could influence decision-making, potentially downplaying the risks associated with certain practices by citing a lack of scientific evidence. It's essential to ensure that academia isn't used solely for bolstering public trust, and decisions shouldn't be solely dictated by market forces (Fox, n.d.).

Analyzing potential conflicts of interest is challenging, especially when considering the partnerships between the AVMA and pharmaceutical companies like Fort Dodge, Merial, and Hill's Pet Nutrition. These companies have collectively committed $4.5 million to support AVMA programs and services over the next four years (Fox, n.d.).

In conclusion, while there are regulations in place for licensing and specialized departments exist on paper, the conflict of interest arising from funding received by these departments from vaccine manufacturers raises significant concerns that warrant careful consideration.

Chapter 6:

Homeopathic Alternatives

to Vaccines

Homeopathy emerged approximately two centuries ago through the pioneering work of Samuel Hahnemann, a German physician. Dr. Hahnemann's exploration began with a curiosity surrounding the effectiveness of quinine in treating malaria. Intrigued, he experimented by ingesting the substance himself and observed that in a healthy individual, it induced symptoms similar to those of malaria. Yet, when administered to a malaria patient, it led to a healing outcome (Pitcairn, n.d.).

Through his investigations, Dr. Hahnemann discovered the principle of "like cures like," wherein substances could prompt healing by mimicking the symptoms of an ailment in a controlled manner. He modified treatments to gently coax the patient's system toward the specific illness, inducing a mild replication of its symptoms (Pitcairn, n.d.). This approach effectively strengthened the body's innate defenses, as if the immune system couldn't tell apart the actual disease from the induced symptoms from a similar substance.

Homeopaths tailor medications to bolster the body's ability to combat illness effectively. They utilize a variety of substances, including herbs and toxins, which are recognized for their influence on the body, emotions, and psyche. These substances undergo meticulous preparation by pharmacists to ensure safety and effectiveness (Pitcairn, n.d.). Through dilution, harmful effects are mitigated while the therapeutic properties are enhanced, often through agitation or grinding. This approach bears similarity to the mechanisms of vaccines and allergy treatments, aiding in the gradual adaptation to harmful agents (Pitcairn, n.d.).

In this chapter, we will explain how homeopathic treatment is different from allopathy, what is the homeopathic alternative to vaccination, the diseases that can be successfully prevented through these alternatives to vaccinations, and finally, we will briefly discuss if the homeopathic alternative can completely replace vaccination in pets.

How Homeopathy Is Different From Allopathy

The term "allopathic" refers to the conventional medical approach that focuses on treating symptoms rather than the disease itself. For instance, if someone has diarrhea, they might be given medicine to slow down their bowels (Pitcairn, n.d.).

On the other hand, homeopathy works on the principle of "like cures like," which means treating a condition with something that produces similar symptoms.

Homeopaths consider two things: what causes the illness (like a germ or toxin) and how the body is reacting to it (like fever or inflammation). While they acknowledge the cause, their main goal is to help the body's natural defenses fight off the illness and heal itself. Their aim is to boost the body's strength and support recovery (Pitcairn, n.d.).

Homeopathy works by using medicines to create a temporary disruption in the body's balance of health. When this disruption is similar to the symptoms caused by the illness, it prompts the body to work harder to recover. The improvements in health that follow are a result of this stimulation. Although the idea is simple, it takes skill and experience to apply, especially for long-term conditions. The homeopathic doctor carefully observes how the body responds to each medicine, guiding the patient through a process of healing that may take weeks or months. During this time, the body fights off the illness and repairs any damaged tissues (Pitcairn, n.d.).

Homeopathic Vaccines: Nosodes

Homeopathic nosodes are often talked about as options instead of regular vaccines. The word comes from the Greek words *nosos* (disease) and *eidos* (like), meaning "like disease." They've been used in homeopathy since the mid-1800s. In veterinary care, they're not very well known and are a hot topic in holistic veterinary communities (Cooney, 2022).

Samuel Hahnemann, who's considered the founder of homeopathy, introduced the idea of nosodes. These are super diluted mixtures made from parts of a disease or infected tissues, used to prevent sickness. Even though both vaccines and nosodes come from diseases, they're quite different.

Unlike vaccines made in labs, nosodes are prepared in a special way. They start with diseased tissues or fluids. Through a process called potentization, the harmful parts get neutralized, and the mix turns into a kind of energetic remedy that works with the body's energy. The end result is a strong remedy that acts like a blueprint of the original disease (Cooney, 2022).

Potentized simply means that the nosode is diluted and shaken repeatedly, just like other homeopathic medicines. Unlike vaccines, nosodes don't contain the disease itself. Instead, they're made by diluting biological material, usually in factors of 100 (Dodds, 2016b).

The idea behind nosodes is that the energy or memory of the disease gets transferred to the diluted mixture. This transfer only happens if the mixture is shaken in a specific way, called succussion. The more the mixture is diluted and succussed, the stronger the nosode becomes (Dodds, 2016b).

To make sure there are no infectious particles left, the dilution of nosodes has to be really high, more than a certain number called Avogadro's number. Some veterinarians practicing conventional medicine fear that although nosodes are safe to use, too much dilution could decrease their effectiveness. They basically believe that nosodes are not likely to cause harm but might not protect against the disease they're meant to (Dodds, 2016b). Holistic Veterinarians argue that the consistent effectiveness of nosodes in preventing diseases reported by the vets who use them refutes the "dilution decrease efficacy" argument (Cooney, 2022).

You take nosodes by mouth. Dr. Charles Loops suggests starting them as early as six weeks old. You give them every two weeks, then every three weeks, and finally once a month. Usually, you can stop giving nosodes when the animal is six months old (Dodds, 2016b).

There are a lot of anecdotal stories from veterinarians, other healthcare workers, and pet owners who use homeopathic nosodes to prevent diseases in animals. They say their animals stay healthy (Dodds, 2016b).

Dr. Jean Dodd argues that although the veterinarians who use nosodes vouch for their effectiveness, there are very few published scientific studies on their effectiveness. Also, vaccines protect against the main virus and can sometimes protect against new versions of it, but nosodes are not known to do that (Dodds, 2016b).

Diseases Successfully Treated With Alternative/Homeopathic Remedies

The main nosodes were tested to see how they worked, just like any other medicine. In veterinary homeopathy, they're used based on the animal's symptoms, matching them to the symptoms the nosode treats (Cooney, 2022).

Later on, in the late 1800s, vets started using nosodes made for specific diseases in animals, like anthrax in cows (called Anthracinum) and distemper in dogs (called Distemperinum) (Cooney, 2022).

Dr. Constantine Hering brought in a nosode called hydrophobinum, made from the saliva of a rabid dog. He used it to treat and prevent rabies in dogs and people. Usually, it's given in 30c potency every few days, and the time between doses increases as the patient gets better. Nowadays, this nosode is known as **lyssin**, and it's often used to help with side effects from the rabies vaccine (Cooney, 2022).

Kennel Cough

Kennel cough is like the common cold for dogs, so it usually only causes mild symptoms and rarely leads to pneumonia. One well-known study about nosodes was done by Christopher Day, a veterinarian who uses homeopathy. There was an outbreak of kennel cough at a dog boarding place in the UK.

In the study, 214 dogs were looked at. Some got a regular vaccine for things like distemper, and others got a vaccine for kennel cough. Some dogs didn't get any vaccines. All dogs were given a 30c dose of nosode twice a day for 3 days.

Before the nosodes, 92.5% of dogs got kennel cough. After the nosodes, only 44.3% got it. This shows a big drop in cases. So, it seems like the kennel cough nosode worked well (Dodds, 2016b).

Distemper

At a city animal shelter, stray dogs were given a nosode for canine distemper to stop the disease from spreading. After they started using the nosode, the percentage of affected dogs dropped from 11.67% to 4.36%, effectively demonstrating the nosode's effectiveness (Dodds, 2016b).

Lepto

In many tropical places, lepto is a big issue, especially during the rainy season. It's a serious illness that can be deadly, with about half of the animals that get it dying from it. Symptoms include fever, abdominal pains, anorexia, diarrhea, abdominal pain, and lethargy.

In Cuba, they used a nosode for lepto, and it helped bring down the fatalities in dogs from the disease (Cooney, 2022).

Dr. Wynn and Dr. Ronald Schultz (University of Wisconsin; Principal Investigator of the Rabies Challenge Fund) gave parvovirus nosode to dogs but reported it failed to provide adequate protection from infection or disease.

Homeopathic Alternatives to Pet Vaccines

Canine Combination Nosode (Hahnemann Labs, California) 200c

This combination nosode includes nosodes to help protect against diseases like distemper, parvo, hepatitis, lepto, kennel cough, and rabies. Many holistic veterinarians have found that giving young puppies one dose of this combination nosode works really well (Cooney, 2022).

The important thing to remember is that nosodes work best when given around the time of possible exposure, like a few days before or after. Most veterinarians suggest using a 30c potency once or twice a week until the puppy is six to eight months old (Cooney, 2022). After that, they might suggest giving nosodes based on the risk of exposure, like if the dog goes to training classes, boarding, grooming, or the dog park.

Since we can't always know when a dog might be exposed to a disease, and nosodes don't seem to give long-lasting protection, veterinaarians recommend giving them regularly until the dog's immune system is strong enough. Usually, by the time a dog reaches puberty, their immune system is good enough, especially if they haven't been vaccinated (Cooney, 2022).

Parvo Nosode 200c

Young puppies seeking protection from Parvovirus are sent home with a small bottle filled with filtered water mixed with parvo nosode 200c and a bit of brandy to keep it preserved (Cooney, 2022). It's suggested to give this mixture to the puppy every week until they're at least six months old. Dr. Ted Cooney, who's been a veterinarian for more than 20 years, says he's never had a puppy die from parvo if they only got nosodes, but some puppies that were also vaccinated did pass away. In his clinic, they noticed that the number of parvo cases went down steadily over three years from 2019 to 2022 (Cooney, 2022).

Heartworm Nosode 30c and 200c

This nosode provides a good option without using drugs or chemicals to strengthen the body's defense against heartworms. Dr. Cooney says he hasn't seen a dog test positive for heartworms while taking the nosode. He's even treated dogs that tested positive previously with heartworm nosodes. He suggests giving either 30c or 200c every one to two weeks during heartworm season, which changes depending on where you live (Cooney, 2022).

After this detailed discussion, you might wonder if nosodes can take the place of vaccines. While the success of nosodes in preventing diseases is apparent to everyone, some veterinarians believe more research is needed to be sure. Because they're safe, effective, and often cheaper, more holistic veterinarians and pet owners are giving nosodes a try.

But for more conservative veterinarians, until more solid studies and feedback from lots of pet owners are made available, nosodes are still a bit of a question mark. They refrain from using them alone to prevent diseases.

All veterinarians, whether practicing homeopathy or allopathy, agree that whenever an alternative to regular medicine is used, it's important to let the pet owner know it's an option that might not be proven. They should give their okay in writing before it is tried (Dodds, 2016b). However, when it comes to the rabies vaccine, it's required by law, so all veterinarians have to follow that rule.

Chapter 7

Homeopathic Clinical Case Stories

Unlike allopathic medicine, which often involves taking drugs repeatedly over a long period, homeopathic veterinarians usually give just one dose of a medication. They choose this medicine based on the animal's current symptoms and their entire medical history. By matching the remedy closely to the animal's overall health picture, they aim to trigger the body's natural healing process. The ultimate aim of homeopathic treatment is to cure the animal without any negative side effects or the need for ongoing medication (Stieg et al., n.d.).

Here are a few cases presented as evidence that homeopathic treatment works well in treating different ailments in pets. In each of these cases, the allopathic treatment was no longer working for the animal; that is why the pet owners gave the homeopathic treatment a chance and they were not disappointed as the animals made a full recovery.

Homeopathic Treatment of *Hemophilia A* in a Kitten

Briar, a male domestic short-haired kitten, was found as a stray when he was only four weeks old. He grew up eating raw food and didn't get any vaccinations. As a kitten, he was lively and played energetically around the house. At seven weeks old, he bled more than usual when tested for FeLV/FIV. When he was six months old, Briar was taken to the vet to be neutered. Before the surgery, blood tests were done, but again, he bled a lot from where the blood was drawn. Despite this, the vet went ahead with the surgery. Afterward, Briar was agitated and bled heavily from the surgery site. The vet tried to stop the bleeding with stitches and Vitamin K1, but it didn't work (Dayton, n.d.).

When Briar's condition became critical, he was taken to Dr. Dayton, a homeopathic veterinarian. Dr. Dayton chose a remedy called **Phosphorus 30c** because it's known for stopping severe bleeding and counteracting the effects of anesthesia. It's also helpful for blood disorders and fits Briar's temperament. After just one dose, Briar's bleeding stopped, and he became calmer. The next day, he was completely fine, and tests confirmed he had hemophilia A. Since then, apart from two doses of Phosphorus, Briar has been healthy with no other medical issues (Dayton, n.d.).

Homeopathic Treatment of

Lymphoma in a Dog

Rosie, a 12-year-old spayed female German Shorthaired Pointer, came to Dr. Cooney's clinic in October 2012, looking very weak and thin. Her abdomen was swollen with fluid, and despite repeated visits to drain it, she only got temporary relief. The day before Dr. Cooney saw Rosie, her local veterinarian gave a grim outlook as she showed signs of lymphoma and suggested taking her to a specialized hospital. Rosie was weak and wobbly, and her abdomen was distended again despite being recently drained. Her gums were pale, and she seemed mentally dull, almost like she had dementia. She wasn't thirsty even in warm weather (Cooney, n.d.).

Dr. Cooney decided to give Rosie a remedy called **Apis mellifica**, which is made from honeybee. It's known for treating symptoms like swollen abdomen, soreness, and lack of thirst. Rosie received one dose of Apis 200c potency (Cooney, n.d.).

Over the next two weeks, Rosie had some good days and some bad ones, but overall, she got better. Her swollen abdomen went down slowly, and she started eating a bit better, though not consistently. Rosie became thirstier than before and seemed a bit grumpier toward other dogs, which was unusual for her. She also got jumpy around loud noises like gunshots (Cooney, n.d.).

Rosie was given a dose of **Nat-m 200c**, known for treating excessive thirst, irritability, and other symptoms.

Within a few days, her appetite and mood started to improve. Three weeks later, she came back for a check-up, and she was back to her normal weight, with good energy. The only lingering issues were increased thirst and occasional bladder leakage while walking. Therefore, she was given a higher dose of Nat-m 1M (Cooney, n.d.).

In January 2014, Rosie's owner reported that she was doing great, running around with other dogs, playing with her grand puppies, and enjoying life (Cooney, n.d.).

Homeopathic Treatment of *Splenic Mass, Persistent Leukocytosis, and Protein Losing Nephropathy* in a Dog

Howie, a 10-year-old neutered male Shih Tzu, had been feeling weak, not eating well, and was diagnosed with anemia. Further tests showed he had masses in his spleen, fluid in his abdomen, and a kidney problem. A specialist suspected leukemia because of these symptoms. Howie was given pain medicine, but it didn't help, so Dr. Melling gave him a homeopathic remedy called **Phosphorus 30c** (Melling, n.d.). His owners were asked to try feeding him homemade food and to let Dr. Melling know how he was doing.

After a few days, Howie started feeling better. His energy improved, and his appetite came back. He was acting more like his usual self, playful and lively. Since then, he's been healthy with no signs of illness (Melling, n.d.). Dr.

Melling continued the treatment based on his blood tests, not because he got worse. His owners are grateful to homeopathy for helping Howie feel better.

Homeopathic Treatment for *Immune-Mediated Polyarthritis*

Treating polyarthritis with homeopathy is a gentle but effective approach aimed at curing the patient. Take the case of a two-year-old male Boxer dog who received all his vaccinations after adoption. However, after the second shot, he developed a big swelling at the injection site, which eventually healed on its own after a month (Stieg et al., n.d.).

In April 2013, the dog's veterinarian noticed swollen joints, crackling sounds in his paws, and suspected immune-mediated polyarthritis—treatment with steroids caused side effects. By August 2013, the symptoms persisted for over five months, prompting the owner to seek homeopathic treatment (Stieg et al., n.d.).

Dr. Stieg selected **Silica** as the remedy because it's known for treating post-vaccination issues, bone diseases, anxiety, and skin problems.

On September 11, 2013, Silica was given to the dog in a single dose of 200C potency. Within the first week, the owner noticed a big improvement in the dog's mood. He seemed happier, walked more comfortably, and started playing with other dogs. After seven days, the owner said he was back to his old self, seeking affection and showing no signs of feeling down (Stieg et al., n.d.).

Three months later, the owner reported that the dog was completely back to normal. He was active, playful, and behaved confidently (Stieg et al., n.d.).

Homeopathy for *Hip Dysplasia:* A Gentle Approach to Chronic Pain

Hip dysplasia is a condition where the hip joint doesn't develop properly, often seen in young dogs. Symptoms can include limping, hopping like a bunny, and weak muscles in the back end. It's usually found in larger dog breeds and can be passed down genetically or influenced by factors like weight.

Merlin, a seven-and-a-half-year-old Border Collie, came to the clinic because his coat was dull and falling out, and his owner was worried it might be a sign of something serious. During the exam, his coat looked dry and thin, his skin was flaky, and he had less muscle in his back legs. He also had trouble moving his hips, especially the right one, and preferred cold places to lie down, which is unusual for dogs with joint problems (Stieg & Melling, n.d.).

Considering Merlin's symptoms, he was given a dose of **Sulphur,** a homeopathic remedy, in 200c potency. Sulfur is known for treating smelly body odors, dry skin, hair loss, and joint pain. It's also helpful for growth issues, which is relevant for hip dysplasia because it involves improper joint development (Stieg & Melling, n.d.).

Five weeks after Merlin's first dose of Sulphur, he was doing better. His coat was softer, and he could move around more easily. But recently, he had been sleeping more and seemed low on energy because of stress at home, like changes in jobs and moving, plus having a dog visitor he didn't get along with. Extreme stress can make a homeopathic remedy less effective, so Merlin got another dose of Sulphur. Three weeks later, he was playful again, waking up easier and seeming happier (Stieg & Melling, n.d.).

Merlin only needed two more doses of Sulphur over the next two years. Each time, his symptoms were milder, showing that the treatment was working well for him (Stieg & Melling, n.d.). He's a great example of how homeopathy can help manage the pain of hip dysplasia effectively.

Summary

Knowing how a disease develops and what makes it dangerous helps us find the best ways to prevent it. Usually, the strongest protection comes from contracting the actual disease and mounting a natural immune response. Vaccines try to copy this natural protection without making the animal go through the illness, although they are not without risks.

Instead of just deciding whether to give vaccines or not, it's better to think about how your pet gets them. Veterinarians strongly recommend not skipping vaccines altogether because pets without them are much more likely to get and spread deadly diseases, with up to 80% dying from them (Becker, 2023a). Pet owners naturally want to keep their pets safe from serious illnesses that could kill them. The tricky part is knowing which vaccines are really necessary and which ones can be skipped, especially for indoor pets.

The first vaccine for dogs was for rabies, and it was made available in the 1920s. Nowadays, it's the only vaccine required by law in many places to protect dogs from rabies (Becker, 2011).

In 1923, a combination vaccine, now called the distemper vaccine, was made to stop common illnesses in dogs like distemper, parvovirus, and hepatitis. Nowadays, there are two main types of vaccines for cats and dogs: core vaccines and non-core vaccines. Core vaccines may be necessary for every pet, while non-core vaccines are given based on their lifestyle and special needs, especially if they might get unusual diseases and need extra protection.

Core vaccines for dogs include shots for distemper, parvovirus, adenovirus, and rabies (AAHA, 2022a).

Core vaccines for cats include shots for panleukopenia, calici, herpes, and rabies (Dodds, 2013).

Research shows that a positive titer test for distemper, parvovirus, and adenovirus indicates strong immunity in dogs (Becker, 2011). It's important to know that while these core vaccines might be required by places like veterinanry clinics or groomers, they're not mandated by the state. Some pet owners worry about legal issues if they don't get vaccines, but in reality, they're not breaking any laws.

Legally, the only vaccine pets must have is for rabies. However, the law usually doesn't recognize a positive titer test for rabies as proof of immunity for pets, just for humans (Becker, 2011). This causes a problem because laws make pet owners and veternarians vaccinate animals over and over, even if they're already immune to rabies. These unnecessary shots don't make immunity stronger and can harm some animals. Recent studies suggest we should reconsider how often we give rabies vaccines (Becker, 2011). The adjuvants in the vaccine that help it work could be toxic, so we might need safer options. We need more research to make rabies vaccines better, with fewer shots and fewer side effects. By keeping up with new discoveries in veterinary science, we can keep our pets healthy and safe.

Vaccines have helped lower the risk of serious diseases, but they can also cause long-lasting health problems. They challenge the body's immune system by putting weakened or dead germs directly into the bloodstream, which can interfere with the immune system and lead to ongoing and chronic health issues in animals. Even though vaccines protect against certain diseases, they might weaken the immune system and bring out other problems like epilepsy, skin allergies, infections, and cancer. Pets today might be feeling the effects of getting too many vaccines over time, known as vaccinosis. (Loops, n.d.).

Because some pets have bad reactions to vaccines and other allopathic medicines, some owners are trying homeopathic treatments. Unlike allopathic medicine, which often requires lots of doses over a long time, homeopathic veterinarians usually give just 1-2 doses. They choose medicines based on the pet's symptoms and medical history to boost the body's natural healing. Homeopathic treatments aim to cure the pet without causing any adverse side effects or needing more medicine later. A simple online search of *"homeopathic veterinarians"* will likely provide many qualified clinics in your area that you can consult with if you need a second opinion, or just want to try a more natural approach to your pet's healthcare.

An important factor in vaccine acceptability is issues related to its licensing. Before a vaccine can be used, it needs approval from the government. This means showing lots of information about how the vaccine is made and tested to make sure it's safe and works well. Approval makes sure the vaccine meets all the rules before it's allowed to be used.

To effectively monitor and address vaccine reactions, as of December 2019, vaccine manufacturers are required to submit all reports of adverse reactions in vaccinated pets to the USDA (Protect The Pets, n.d.). Pet owners should also report any adverse reactions to the USDA.

Both pet owners and veterinarians need to be concerned about vaccine safety because reactions can happen immediately or later on. If you suspect an adverse reaction, report it and provide all the requested information to help make changes. It's a legal requirement to get your pet's medical records, so ask for them as soon as you suspect a reaction. Important information to gather from the records includes the vaccine brand, serial number, and expiration date.

Here's a cheat sheet to help you report:

- Gather your records.

- Report online or by calling.

- Share your report on social media to encourage others.

- Email your State Veterinary Board if you weren't told about the risks or if they ignored the reaction.

When reporting, provide information about the animal, the event, and the product used. Include details like the animal's species, breed, age, and weight. Also, provide your contact information and details about the adverse event, such as when it happened and how long it lasted. Include information about the vaccine, like its brand and expiration date. Make sure to mention if the product was used correctly according to the label instructions. If you need help, you can call the USDA, but ask them to send you a copy of your report.

References

American Animal Hospital Association (AAHA). (2022a). . AAHA.org https://www.aaha.org/aaha-guidelines/2022-aaha-canine-vaccination-guidelines/faqs/

American Animal Hospital Association (AAHA). (2022b). *Vaccine licensure.* AAHA.org https://www.aaha.org/aaha-guidelines/2022-aaha-canine-vaccination-guidelines/vaccine-licensure/

American Veterinary Medical Association (AVMA). (n.d.). *Vaccinations.* AVMA.org. https://www.avma.org/resources-tools/pet-owners/petcare/vaccinations

Becker, K. (2011, May 31) *How often should you vaccinate your cat or dog.* Barks & Whiskers. https://www.barkandwhiskers.com/2011-05-31-nl-what-your-vet-didnt-tell-you-about-all-those-puppy-and-kitty-vaccines/

Becker, K. (2018, December 5). *Two big, common mistakes made with rabies vaccine.* Barkes & Whiskers. https://www.barkandwhiskers.com/2018-12-05-nl-rabies-virus-vaccine/

Becker, K. (2021 July 10). *Study shows rabies vaccine is effective for at least 5 years.* Barks & Whiskers.

https://www.barkandwhiskers.com/2021-07-10-nl-5-year-rabies-vaccine/

Becker, K. (2022, November 22). *What you need to know about vaccinating your cat.* Barkes & Whiskers. https://www.barkandwhiskers.com/feline-vaccination-guidelines/

Becker, K. (2023a, February 12). *How to protect your pet from vaccine damage.* Barkes & Whiskers. https://www.barkandwhiskers.com/what-is-vaccinosis/

Becker, K. (2023b, May 22). *Why I don't recommend non-core canine vaccines.* Barkes & Whiskers. https://www.barkandwhiskers.com/canine-vaccination/

Becker, K. (2023c, October 23). *How long do vaccines really last?* Barkes & Whiskers. https://www.barkandwhiskers.com/2023-10-23-canine-titers/

Becker, K. & Schultz, R. (2014). *Does your pet really need that rabies shot?* Protect The Pets. https://www.protectthepets.com/uploads/1/0/8/0/108023613/does_your_pet_really_need_that_rabies_shot_-_schultz__2014__transcript_of_4_part_video_series.pdf

Burakova, Y., Madera, R., McVey, S., Schlup, J. R., & Shi, J. (2018). Adjuvants for animal vaccines. *Viral Immunology, 31*(1), 11–22. https://doi.org/10.1089/vim.2017.0049

Cooney, T. (n.d.). *Homeopathic treatment of lymphoma in a dog, a curative case.* Pitcairn Institute of Veterinary Homeopathy. https://pivh.org/sfd/library/library-examples-2/homeopathic-treatment-of-lymphoma-in-a-dog-a-curative-case-todd-cooney-dvm-cvh/

Cooney, T. (2022, August 10). Immunity and homeopathy in dogs — focus on nosodes. *Innovative Veterinary Journal.* https://ivcjournal.com/immunity-and-homeopathy-in-dogs-focus-on-nosodes/

Children's Health Defence Team. (2021, June 25). *Dog doc' Marty Goldstein tells RFK Jr. about holistic pet care + Harms of over vaccinating.* https://childrenshealthdefense.org/defender/marty-goldstein-rfk-jr-the-defender-podcast-holistic-pet-care-vaccinating/

Cromwell, J (n.d.). *James Cromwell quotes.* BrainyQuote. https://www.brainyquote.com/quotes/james_cromwell_389786

Dayton, S. (n.d.). *Homeopathic treatment of hemophilia A in a kitten.* Pitcairn Institute of Veterinary Homeopathy. https://pivh.org/sfd/library/library-examples-2/homeopathic-treatment-of-hemophilia-a-in-a-kitten-by-siri-dayton-dvm/

Dodds, J. (2013, November 13). Feline vaccination protocol. *Dr. Jean Dodds' Pet Health Resource Blog.* https://drjeandoddspethealthresource.tumblr.c

om/post/66885321280/dodds-cat-vaccination-protocol-2013-2014

Dodds, J. (2016a, July 10). Nosodes instead of vaccines. *Dr. Jean Dodds' Pet Health Resource Blog.* https://drjeandoddspethealthresource.tumblr.com/post/147197863796/nosodes-vs-vaccines#.WOQ3ym8rK1u

Dodds, J. (2016b, July 18). Dodds vaccination protocol for dogs. *Dr. Jean Dodds' Pet Health Resource Blog.* https://drjeandoddspethealthresource.tumblr.com/post/147595920886/dodds-vaccination-protocol-dogs-2016#.V4zv87grLIU

Driscoll, C. (2021, December 15) *The purdue vaccination studies and auto-antibodies.* Dogs Naturally Magazine. https://www.dogsnaturallymagazine.com/purdue-vaccination-studies/

European Advisory Board on Cat Diseases (ABCD Europe). (2022, June 23). *Vaccines and vaccination, an introduction.* ABCD Cats Vets. https://www.abcdcatsvets.org/vaccines-and-vaccination-an-introduction/

Fox, M. (n.d.). *Conflicts of Interest in the Veterinary Profession.* Encyclopedia Britannica. https://www.britannica.com/explore/savingearth/conflicts-of-interest-in-the-veterinary-profession

Loops, C. (n.d.). *Vaccination information.* Charles Loops DVM.
https://www.charlesloopsdvm.com/vacc-info

McVey, Scott. & Shi, Jishu. (2010, May 13). *Vaccines in veterinary medicine: A brief review of history and technology.* National Library of Medicine.
https://www.ncbi.nlm.nih.gov/pmc/articles/PMC7124274/

Melling, L. (n.d.). *Homeopathic treatment of splenic mass, persistent leukocytosis, and protein losing nephropathy in a dog.* Pitcairn Institute of Veterinary Homeopathy.
https://pivh.org/sfd/library/library-examples-2/homeopathic-treatment-of-splenic-mass-persistent-leukocytosis-and-protein-losing-nephro/

O'Niell, F. (n.d.). *A history of rabies.* Tuckahoe Veterinary Hospital.
https://www.tuckahoevet.com/post/a-history-of-rabies

Pitcairn, R. (n.d.). *Homeopathy: A science explained.* Pitcairn Institute of Veterinary Homeopathy.
https://pivh.org/sfd/what-is-homeopathy/

Roth, J., Brown G., & Flaming, K. (n.d.). *Principles of veterinary vaccinology.* The Centre for Food Security & Public Health.
https://www.cfsph.iastate.edu/Assets/SampleVaccOutline.pdf

Preventative medicine: Feline injection-site sarcoma. (2013, July/August). Today's Veterinary Practice

(TVP).
https://todaysveterinarypractice.com/preventiv
e-medicine/feline-injection-site-sarcoma/

Purdue University. (n.d.). *Immune-mediated diseases.*
https://vet.purdue.edu/hospital/small-
animal/resources/immune-mediated-
diseases.php

Schultz, R. (2016, February 5). *Dr. Schultz letter of support.*
Protect The Pets.
https://www.protectthepets.com/uploads/1/0
/8/0/108023613/dr._r_schultz_feb_2016_lette
r_of_support_edited_with_permission.pdf

The science has been done. (2003). Critter Advocacy
Organization (CAO).
https://www.protectthepets.com/uploads/1/0
/8/0/108023613/the_science_has_been_done.
pdf

Stieg, S. & Melling, L. (n.d.). *Homeopathy for hip dysplasia:
A gentle approach to chronic pain.* Pitcairn Institute
of Veterinary Homeopathy.
https://pivh.org/sfd/library/library-examples-
2/homeopathic-treatment-of-hip-displasia-in-a-
dog-by-sarah-stieg-dvm-mrcvs-and-lisa-melling-
dvm-cvh/

Stieg, S., Melling, L., & Cooney, T. (n.d.). *Homeopathic
treatment for immune-mediated polyarthritis.* Pitcairn
Institute of Veterinary Homeopathy.
https://pivh.org/sfd/library/homeopathic-
treatment-for-immune-mediated-polyarthritis-

by-sarah-stieg-dvm-mrcvs-lisa-melling-dvm-
cvh-and-todd-cooney-dvm-cvh/

Take Action – Report Reactions! Protect The Pets. (n.d.).
https://www.protectthepets.com/uploads/1/0
/8/0/108023613/vaaeblog.pdf

Tizard, I. & Payne, S. (2011, July). *Vaccines and
immunotherapy.* MSD Veterinary Manual.
https://www.msdvetmanual.com/special-pet-
topics/drugs-and-vaccines/vaccines-and-
immunotherapy

Veterinary biologic. (n.d.). ScienceDirect.
https://www.sciencedirect.com/topics/veterina
ry-science-and-veterinary-medicine/veterinary-
biologic

Williams, K., Ward, E., & Gollakner, R. (n.d.-a). *Vaccines
for cats.* VCA Animal Hospitals.
https://vcahospitals.com/know-your-
pet/vaccines-for-cats

Williams, K., Ward, E., & Gollakner, R. (n.d.-b). *Vaccines
for dogs.* VCA Animal Hospitals.
https://vcahospitals.com/know-your-
pet/vaccines-for-dogs

Yale, G., Sudarshan, S., Taj, S., Patchimuthu, G.,
Mangalanathan, B., Belludi, A., Shampur, M.,
Krishnaswamy, T., & Mazeri, S. (2021, April 5).
*Investigation of protective level of rabies antibodies in
vaccinated dogs in Chennai, India.* National Library
of   Medicine.
https://www.ncbi.nlm.nih.gov/pmc/articles/P
MC8110021/

www.ingramcontent.com/pod-product-compliance
Lightning Source LLC
Chambersburg PA
CBHW070811260726

48660CB00005B/1815